Preventive
Primary Medicine

D0964266

Preventive Primary Medicine

Reducing the Major Causes of Mortality

Robert Lewy, M.D., M.P.H.

*Adjunct Assistant Professor of Public Health
and Associate Physician Medical Service,
Columbia University College of Physicians and Surgeons*

*Director, Employee Health Service,
The Presbyterian Hospital in the City of New York*

Little, Brown and Company
Boston

To my parents

Foreword

The promise of preventive medicine is in the air, the same air that surrounds and sustains our patients as well as ourselves, but few of our patients share their physicians' sober recognition of the limits of prevention. This "reality gap" defines the need for a great deal more health education than has been made available to overexpectant patients.

Preventive medicine has been greatly oversold to the American public by legislators and other politicians, by feature-hungry editors of newspapers and lay magazines, by vendors of vitamins and other drugs, by entrepreneurs who operate spas and fitness centers—and, yes, by some few physicians, nurses, and other health-care "providers," well intentioned or otherwise. At the same time, preventive medicine has been almost uniformly undersold to physicians by their medical schools and hospitals wherein care of the esoterically or critically ill patient is emphasized. Most important, prevention has been given short shrift by those in the best position to influence health care, namely the fiscal intermediaries (commercial and government) who pay for what patients get.

Should your patients worry about their weight, their food, their drink? Should they quit smoking? Could they? How? Is it true what they say about cholesterol? Can they "fight cancer with a checkup"? Is jogging worthwhile?

While doctors and nurses have been too busy and too few to hear these questions, the answers have been provided to patients by fundraisers, advertisers, and tellers of old wives' tales. With renewed emphasis on primary care by the greater numbers of health professionals being pumped into a stabilizing national population, our patients will expect more reasoned responses from more legitimate medical spokespeople.

It is to these primary care–oriented physicians, nurses, and students that Dr. Lewy addresses this book. Trained in internal medicine and board-certified in family medicine, Dr. Lewy has practiced preventive primary medicine in locations as disparate as an American Indian reservation in the Southwest, a New England hamlet in northernmost Vermont, and an Ivy League university–affiliated hospital in Manhattan. He has subjected this hands-on experience to the statistical and other analytical techniques learned en route to an M.P.H. degree, then reviewed the product in the context of the medical literature. The distillate is in your hands, and I share his hope that it will help you to help your patients become more effective participants in the maintenance of their own health and well-being.

John L. Roglieri, M.D.

Assistant Professor of Clinical Medicine, Columbia University College of Physicians and Surgeons

Vice-President, Ambulatory Services, The Presbyterian Hospital in the City of New York

Preface

The underlying premise of this book is that reductions in the leading causes of mortality in the United States will not occur through advances in curative treatment as rapidly as through advances in early disease detection and preventive education. Progress in earlier detection of disease and in preventive education can occur most readily through the diligent and aggressive application of preventive measures by primary care physicians. Preventive medicine should and undoubtedly will play an increasing role in primary care practice.

Preventive Primary Medicine should serve as an aid in applying known principles of preventive medicine in primary care practice. I hope that it will provide a data base and adequate guidelines for the development and implementation of a personalized patient-screening program for the leading causes of mortality.

The book is organized into 10 chapters, each dealing with a major cause of mortality. Each chapter follows a similar format and covers occurrence, etiology, risk factors, screening, prevention, and summary and recommendations. The 15 leading causes of mortality in the United States are listed in the table on page x. The 10 causes of mortality discussed in this book account for 84 percent of all deaths in the United States and represent conditions the

*Death Rates from 15 Leading Causes of Death
in the United States in 1975*

Rank	Cause of Death	Death Rate per 100,000	Percent of Total Deaths
1	Diseases of heart	339.0	37.8
2	Malignant neoplasms	174.4	19.5
3	Cerebrovascular diseases	91.8	10.2
4	Accidents	47.6	5.3
5	Influenza & pneumonia	27.0	3.0
6	Diabetes mellitus	16.8	1.9
7	Cirrhosis of liver	15.1	1.7
8	Arteriosclerosis	13.7	1.5
9	Certain causes of mortality in early infancy	12.8	1.4
10	Suicide	12.6	1.4
11	Bronchitis, emphysema, & asthma	11.9	1.3
12	Homicide	10.2	1.1
13	Congenital anomalies	6.7	0.7
14	Nephritis & nephrosis	3.9	0.4
15	Peptic ulcer	3.2	0.4

Source: Vital Statistics Report, Annual Summary for the U.S., 1975, National Center for Health Statistics. Government Printing Office, Washington, D.C., 1976.

prevention of which could have a significant impact in reducing mortality.

Much of the material covered in this book remains controversial. There is as yet no universally accepted preventive health protocol. Although many may not agree with
my specific recommendations, the recommendations are
based on an adequate body of literature. They are not
meant to be dogmatic but merely to serve as guidelines.
Newer studies will, undoubtedly, cause many of the recommendations to be altered.

I hope that having gathered into a single volume information on prevention previously available only from a wide
variety of sources will facilitate the implementation of preventive medicine into primary care practice.

I would like to thank Dr. John Roglieri and Dr. Michael
Stewart, co-Directors of the Clinical Scholar Program at
Columbia University College of Physicians and Surgeons,
for their advice and support during preparation of the
manuscript. I also thank Judy Golden for her excellent
artwork.

R.L.

Contents

Preventive
Primary Medicine

Introduction

Historical Perspectives

Preventive medicine in the United States is in a state of transition, largely because of the changing character of the health problems prevalent. In the early part of the twentieth century, the most pressing health problems were communicable diseases. In 1900, influenza, pneumonia, tuberculosis, and infections of the gastrointestinal tract accounted for one-third of all deaths. Typhoid fever and malaria outbreaks were relatively common; diphtheria was the tenth leading cause of death and a major source of mortality among children. Measles, pertussis, scarlet fever, rheumatic fever, meningococcal infections, and syphilis were common sources of illness and death.

Nutritional and environmentally related diseases were also rampant at that time. Fifty to 80 percent of children seen in clinics had signs of rickets. The death rate for diarrhea hovered at 23 deaths per 1,000. Illness and death among pregnant women were common, since prenatal care was nonexistent and many women delivered babies without medical supervision.

During this period, public health maintained distinct boundaries from the clinical practice of medicine. This distinction arose from the emphasis of public health prac-

1

titioners on problems and populations that were not ordinarily dealt with by private practitioners. Local and state health departments, with support from the federal government, provided for the collection and analysis of vital statistics, control of communicable diseases, sanitation, food and milk control, laboratory services, public health nursing and education, and maternal, infant, and child health care for those who had no access to a private practitioner.

While the health departments were concerned with the community and with health services, clinical practitioners remained oriented to individual patients and to the diagnosis and treatment of disease. Private practice was organized to treat episodes of illness, so disease prevention and health maintenance did not readily fit into the usual practice pattern. The concept of prevention through community action had little relevance to the private practitioner, who was content to have the health department provide such services.

In the latter half of this century, as the morbidity and mortality from communicable diseases decreased, the increasing numbers of survivors reached older age and chronic degenerative diseases became increasingly prevalent. Preventive medicine had to expand to include control of these chronic diseases as well as communicable diseases. The involvement of health practitioners in chronic disease control led to the dissolution of the traditional division between prevention as practiced by public health specialists and cure as practiced by private physicians. Prevention became of increasing concern to private as well as public health practitioners.

Implementing Prevention into Clinical Practice

While the importance of prevention in reducing morbidity and mortality has become generally accepted, the incorporation of prevention into clinical practice remains one of the greatest challenges to modern health care. Despite the acceptance of the theories of preventive medicine, there remain obstacles in their application. The organization and financing of health care have been largely responsible for discouraging the incorporation of prevention into clinical practice. Specialization and practice habits that emphasize the episodic care of illness have deemphasized the importance of preventive medical care. Reimbursement mechanisms that do not allow physicians to bill for many preventive services virtually insure the secondary role of prevention.

The specialty of preventive medicine has never achieved the professional status of other medical specialties. As long as the financial rewards of clinical practice continue to outweigh the financial rewards of preventive practice, preventive medicine will continue to be a minor specialty. Nor has preventive medicine ever been a popular subject among medical students or clinicians. In 1953, J.M. MacKintosh, Professor of Public Health at the University of London, observed [1]:

> *Everyone says that prevention is better than cure, and hardly anyone acts as if he believes it . . . palliatives nearly always take precedence over prevention, and our health services today are too heavily loaded with salvage. Treatment, the attempt to heal the sick, is more tangible, more exciting and more immediately rewarding than prevention.*

There are, however, some encouraging trends emerging in the primary care movement. The primary care physician, by assuming responsibility for comprehensive rather than only episodic care, has a greater opportunity to practice preventive medicine. The new specialty of family practice, for example, has made a bold commitment to preventive medicine. Screening, health maintenance, and health education are recognized concerns of the family practitioner. Family practice residents are required to obtain training in community medicine, the study of the health of a defined population.

Preventive medicine can be effectively practiced only if patients have a positive attitude toward the concept. Since much of prevention requires an asymptomatic person to modify his life-style, the individual must be suitably motivated to do so. Unlike curative medicine, rapid and dramatic changes do not occur. Thus, in order for a patient to continue practicing prevention, he must receive continued follow-up and reinforcement. Group or peer pressure can provide some motivation and reinforcement.

The primary care physician, by virtue of his ongoing, comprehensive relationship with the patient, can also suitably motivate and reinforce the patient to act preventively. If the patient feels the physician is willing to accept continuing and comprehensive responsibility for maintaining his health, he may be more willing to accept preventive recommendations.

When the primary physician recommends a preventive program, that program should be individualized to deal with the patient's particular problems and needs. An authoritarian, standard warning will rarely produce lasting results.

Before any change in attitude or behavior can occur, the patient must understand the risks involved for himself. He should be informed about how occupational hazards, smoking, diet, or exercise habits, for example, may relate to increased health risks. The patient should also be taught how he can increase the chances of early detection through screening tests or by performing simple self-examinations. Only when the patient understands the risks and how to decrease them, can the physician expect any compliance. It is the responsibility of the primary care physician, or his assistant, to educate and motivate his patients to reduce risks.

Another important feature of the practice of preventive medicine is patient recall and follow-up. Preventive care, unlike episodic care, requires more than just waiting for patients to present their complaints. Proper preventive care should include a recall system to monitor patients periodically.

Primary care physicians maintain a continual relationship with patients. They are familiar with their patients' social and occupational environments and are responsible for integrating all aspects of health and medical care. Primary care physicians are thus in an ideal position to implement prevention into their clinical practice. This can readily be done by

1. Identifying high-risk individuals
2. Screening the population at risk
3. Detecting disease in its earliest stages
4. Providing health education for primary prevention
5. Identifying and participating in efforts to remove harmful agents from the workplace and the ambient environment

Screening

Although screening and the identification of high-risk groups have traditionally been the function of public health specialists, primary care physicians are in a particularly advantageous position to intercede by viewing the leading causes of mortality as personal health as well as public health problems. The interests and skills of the primary care physician in health maintenance, health screening, and preventive medicine can act as a vital link between public health and the practice of clinical medicine.

Screening sorts out apparently well persons who may have a disease from those who probably do not. Screening is intended to identify unrecognized disease through the use of procedures and tests that can be economically and rapidly performed. Although screening can be applied to large, asymptomatic populations, it has proved to be most effective when selectively directed at individuals in high-risk categories. Selective screening has far greater cost-effectiveness and potential rewards than the indiscriminate application of tests to large groups of people.

Risk factors are important in identifying the distribution of a disease in a population. In order to apply rational selective screening procedures, the primary care physician must be able to identify high-risk individuals. Selective screening not only increases the efficiency and yield of screening, but also decreases unnecessary patient discomfort, cost, and hazards. Risk factors can be identified by

1. Age, sex, and race
2. Signs and symptoms
3. Personal and medical history
4. Environment and occupation

Selective screening requires that the primary care physician develop a comprehensive patient data base determined by known risk factors. Since 70 percent of patients see their primary care physician at least once a year, the most economical way of applying selective screening is within the context of regular, ongoing care.

Mass screening has received enthusiastic support, especially from prepaid health plans. However, when it is subject to critical analysis, there seems to be little justification for its use. Many times indiscriminate screening procedures detect diseases for which there may be no treatment or where early diagnosis has no benefit to the patient. The following principles of screening are well-accepted criteria by which to judge the worth of a procedure [2]. These criteria can be aptly applied to the screening procedures covered in the following chapters of the book.

1. The problem must be important, i.e., it must be of significance to the individual and detrimental to health if left untreated.
2. Effective treatment must be available. There is no need to identify a disease for which no treatment exists.

3. Treatment should be accessible. Persons found in need of treatment should have treatment facilities available.
4. The test and treatment must be acceptable to the patient. Screening tests should be easy and quick to perform and present mimimal discomfort to the patient. The patient should also be willing to undergo the treatment for the disease.
5. Early detection should be advantageous. Early diagnosis should lead to more efficient treatment and a better prognosis.
6. The course and natural history of the disease should be understood. There should exist a latent and early symptomatic phase that could warrant detection during this period.
7. The condition should either have some prevalence in the community or be especially serious.
8. Tests should be sufficiently sensitive and specific. There should be few false negative and false positive results.
9. Disease identification should be cost-effective. The cost of detecting a case must be reasonable in relation to the individual and the community.

Because of the changing nature of our prevalent health problems, preventive medicine will assume an increasingly important role in medical care practice. The primary care physician is in an ideal position to incorporate preventive medicine techniques into daily practice. If these techniques are applied in a rational manner, they could have a significant effect in decreasing mortality.

References

1. MacKintosh, J.M *Trends of Opinion About the Public Health 1901-1951.* Oxford University Press, London, 1953. P. 5.
2. Wilson, J.M., and G. Junger. *Principles and Practice of Screening for Disease.* World Health Organization Press, Geneva, 1968.

1

Arteriosclerotic Cardiovascular Disease

Occurrence

Coronary heart disease (CHD) is this country's most important health problem, not only because of its magnitude, but also because much of it could be prevented. With the second highest death rate from CHD in the world, men in the United States have one chance in three of developing some form of symptomatic arterial disease and one chance in five of developing clinical CHD, mostly in the form of acute myocardial infarction, before age 60. Every year one million persons will have an acute myocardial infarction. Of these, 25 percent will die within 3 hours of the onset of symptoms, usually outside of the hospital. An additional 10 percent will die within weeks after the attack. Survivors are five times as likely to die in the next 5 years as those without a prior attack [14].

Diseases of the heart remain the leading cause of death in the United States, accounting for 37.8 percent of all deaths. There are, however, recent indications that the sharp rise in incidence that occurred over the past 40 years may be lessening. Between 1950 and 1975, the age-adjusted death rate from diseases of the heart decreased by 28 percent from 307.6 deaths per 100,000 in 1950 to 222.5 deaths per 100,000 in 1975. The drop was steepest in recent years,

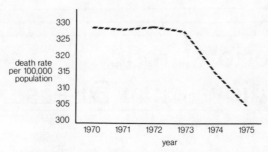

*Figure 1-1. Death rate by year from ischemic
heart disease.*

amounting to 15 percent between 1969 and 1975 (Fig.
1-1).

In view of what is known about the underlying disease
process of CHD, late intervention cannot be expected to
inhibit morbidity and mortality significantly. The exis-
tence of coronary care units during the last 10 years has
contributed relatively little to decreasing total mortality.
Likewise, although coronary artery surgery may prolong
life, a coronary bypass certainly will not change the underlying atherosclerotic disease process. Major progress in controlling CHD is possible, however, through prevention.

Risk Factors

Although the exact pathogenesis of CHD remains obscure,
a large body of laboratory, epidemiological, and clinical
research has identified certain risk factors associated with
its development [13, 20]. Environmental factors are largely
responsible, as indicated by an increasing incidence of
CHD among younger men, by a wide variation in the prevalence of CHD between different countries and between
different regions of the same country, by the development
of CHD in migrants from poor to more affluent countries,
and by the wartime decline of CHD in food-starved countries [17].

Coronary heart disease begins early in life. Intimal thickening of the coronary arteries by an accumulation of lipids, mostly cholesterol, progresses through a latent period until it produces clinical manifestations in middle life. The sudden onset of crushing chest pain, shock, pulmonary edema, or ventricular fibrillation merely reflects the ischemic complications of long existent and severe atherosclerosis. Coronary heart disease can be detected earlier in its course by a coronary risk profile. It is generally accepted that CHD is a multifactorial condition for which risk factors have been identified. Not all risk factors, however, are of equivalent importance among particular population groups or individuals.

A diet habitually high in saturated fats and cholesterol, hypercholesterolemia, hypertension, and cigarette smoking are the major etiologically significant risk factors for CHD. The presence of only one of the major risk factors, as compared to none, is associated with an almost 100 percent increase in risk for a coronary event occurring over the next decade. When combinations of risk factors are present, the risk increases to four or five times that for a similar population with none of the risk factors. Clinical diabetes mellitus, asymptomatic hyperglycemia, obesity, sedentary living, psychosocial stress, and a family history of CHD are risk factors of somewhat less etiological significance.

AGE

The death rate from CHD increases progressively with age (Fig. 1-2).

SEX

Twice as many men as women will develop cardiovascular disease by age 65, and four times as many men as women will die of cardiovascular disease by age 65.

HYPERTENSION

Hypertension is known to accelerate the atherosclerotic process, particularly in combination with hyperlipidemia

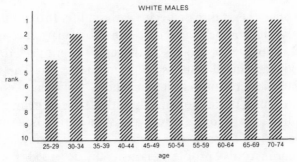

Figure 1-2. Rank of arteriosclerotic heart disease as cause of death by age.

[3]. A substantial number of experimental, clinical, and prospective epidemiological studies have demonstrated a linear relationship between the height of the blood pressure and the risk of CHD. In the VA Cooperative Drug Study, 380 hypertensive men were randomly assigned to either a treatment or a placebo group. Over a 5-year period, the risk of morbidity decreased from 55 to 18 percent for the treatment group. Major cardiovascular events occurred in 35 men of the control group versus 9 men of the treatment group. Although treatment was most effective in preventing congestive heart failure and strokes, and least effective in preventing manifestations of coronary atherosclerosis, recent data support the view that drug treatment of hypertension is effective in preventing CHD.

Hypertension is an exceedingly common condition with its own set of risk factors [3, 11]. Age, sex, race, obesity, and possibly, according to one recent report, alcohol consumption have been associated with hypertension [15]. The prevalence of hypertension increases with age. It is estimated that 15 percent of all white adults and 30 percent of all black adults are hypertensive.

In contrast to the amount of attention focused on hypertension in adults, little is known about the diagnosis, criteria, incidence, and natural history of hypertension in

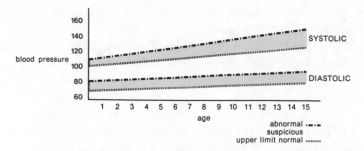

Figure 1-3. Age-related changes in blood pressure in childhood. (From Gruskin [10].)

children. From birth through age 15, there is a steady increase in systolic and diastolic readings (Fig. 1-3). Defining hypertension as greater than 2 standard deviations above the mean, one survey of 1,795 children found that 2.3 percent of children between ages 4 and 15 and 1.4 percent of children between ages 12 and 21 were hypertensive [9]. Unlike adults, in whom 90 percent of hypertension is essential, only 20 percent of children had essential hypertension.

Abundant evidence exists that obesity has a direct positive correlation with blood pressure levels. In addition, many studies have demonstrated that a decrease in weight is associated with a decrease in blood pressure. It has been estimated that control of obesity among the white population in the United States could reduce the prevalence of hypertension by 50 percent. Since it is commonly believed that the fall in blood pressure with weight loss is entirely due to a reduction in salt intake, many experts have tended to neglect the value of weight reduction alone in treating hypertension. In fact, a report of the Joint National Committee on Detection, Evaluation and Treatment of High Blood Pressure minimized the role of weight control in treating hypertension. The committee concluded that weight control may be beneficial to persons with borderline hypertension, but it was not necessarily recommended as part of a treatment program for those with diastolic pressures above 104 mm Hg.

Until recently it has been impossible to separate the effects of weight loss from the effects of salt intake in the treatment of hypertension. However, the results of one study that attempted to evaluate the effect of weight loss on hypertension, while maintaining the same salt intake, indicated that weight loss leads to a decrease in blood pressure independently of salt intake [17]. Weight control seems to offer a safe, low-cost means of blood pressure control. If overweight, hypertensive patients could control their weight, their medication dosages might be lowered or eliminated. A major problem, however, is patient compliance with a dietary program. Nevertheless, weight reduction should be recommended as an initial step and as part of a program of continued treatment for overweight hypertensives.

HYPERLIPIDEMIA

Population studies have shown that there are close links between hyperlipidemia, atherosclerosis, CHD, and diet. Experimental, clinical, and epidemiological studies indicate that hyperlipidemia, influenced by diet, has a high association with and may be a causal factor of CHD. Because of methodological flaws, the crucial and conclusive evidence that the incidence and mortality of CHD can be decreased by dietary means alone is currently not available. It is known, however, that increasing serum cholesterol increases the risk of developing CHD. Recent clinical studies using angiography to assess narrowing of coronary arteries have strengthened the evidence of an association between serum lipid levels and CHD. Patients with narrowing of coronary arteries had increased cholesterol levels compared to patients without such narrowing. The evidence for linking diet to hyperlipidemia as a risk factor is based on the following [20]:

1. CHD is rare among populations with low mean plasma cholesterol levels.
2. CHD at a young age is common in patients with familial hyperlipidemia.
3. There is an approximately linear relationship between plasma cholesterol levels greater than 200 mg/100 ml and the incidence of CHD.
4. Hypertriglyceridemia is probably an independent risk factor.
5. Plasma lipids are mainly derived from foods; thus, plasma lipid levels can be raised or lowered by changes in eating habits.
6. The hallmark of atherosclerotic plaque is the accumulation of cholesterol in it.
7. The concentration of cholesterol in the arterial wall is in proportion to that in the plasma.
8. Atherosclerosis has been induced in primates by their being fed Western-type diets.
9. Pathological changes in experimental animals regress with a reversion to their natural diet.
10. In man, there is a regression of the cutaneous manifestations of hypercholesterolemia after diet or drug therapy to lower hypercholesterolemia.

SMOKING

The 1964 Surgeon General's Report on Smoking established that cigarette smokers have a 70-percent greater chance of developing CHD than nonsmokers. Mortality from CHD increases with the intensity of smoking. Young men who smoke two or more packs of cigarettes per day are at highest risk. Recent work has implicated carbon monoxide in the development of CHD in smokers. Carbon monoxide induces hypoxia, increases endothelial permeability, and may enhance atherosclerosis. Smokers with carboxyhemoglobin levels greater than 5 percent have more than 20 times the incidence of CHD than those with levels below 3 percent. Smokers who change to cigarettes with less tar and nicotine have lower carboxyhemoglobin levels. (See Chap. 3 for a discussion of smoking cessation.)

DIABETES MELLITUS AND ASYMPTOMATIC HYPERGLYCEMIA

Clinical diabetes mellitus has long been recognized as a risk factor for atherosclerotic disease. Retrospective studies have shown that diabetics have atherosclerotic disease more often, more severely, and more prematurely than do nondiabetics. Retrospective studies also indicate that persons with manifestations of atherosclerotic disease have abnormalities in glucose tolerance more often than those in control groups do. Prospective studies indicate that asymptomatic hyperglycemia is an independent risk factor for atherosclerotic disease. The crucial and conclusive evidence that lowering blood sugar will prevent or retard the development of atherosclerosis is lacking, however.

PSYCHOSOCIAL TENSIONS

Despite the unevenness of the quality of research methods and the content of the findings relating psychosocial characteristics to CHD, it is generally accepted that disturbing emotions, anxiety, depression, psychophysiological complaints, general nervousness, and type A behavior patterns (intense striving for achievement, competitive, easily provoked, impatient, sense of time urgency, abrupt speech and gesture, overcommitted to vocation, excess drive, and hostility) are consistently related to the risk of developing coronary disease [10]. Chronic conflict and work overload may also be related but with less strength and consistency. Social variables such as mobility and life changes are even less consistently and less strongly associated with the risk of CHD. It has been hypothesized that the association between CHD and stress is due to excess catecholamine secretion, which results in increased blood pressure, heart rate, circulating lipids, and platelet aggregation.

SEDENTARY LIVING

Epidemiological studies suggest that exercise may have a beneficial effect in decreasing the incidence, severity, and

morbidity of CHD. To assess the role of physical activity
in reducing coronary mortality, one study followed 6,351
longshoremen for 22 years [13]. Work activity was categorized as high, medium, or low in caloric output. The
age-adjusted coronary death rate for the high-activity cate-
gory was 26.9 coronary deaths per 10,000 work years
compared to medium and low categories in which there
were 46.3 and 49.0 coronary deaths per 10,000 work years,
respectively. These findings demonstrate that vigorous
physical exercise is associated with a decreased risk of coronary death.

Another report demonstrated that heart attack rates
were twice as high among Harvard graduates who expended less than 500 cal of exercise per week than among
those who expended more than 2,000 cal of exercise per
week.

Several hypotheses may explain the protective effect of
physical activity on coronary mortality. Conditioning of
the cardiovascular system may prevent or diminish the
chain that starts with ventricular ectopic beats and leads to
fibrillation and death. Another explanation is that high
levels of energy expenditure increase fibrinolytic activity
and decrease platelet aggregation, resulting in decreased
thrombus formation. In addition, increased collateral circulation and increased luminal area of the coronary arteries
result from high energy output. High work output also
decreases the influence of such risk factors as hypertension, hyperlipidemia, obesity, and tachycardia.

Prevention

Research in the past 25 years has contributed much to the
understanding of the epidemiology of CHD. Although the
major risk factors associated with CHD have been identified, the implementation of public and individual preventive programs has been controversial. Two major criticisms

have impeded the widespread application of primary preventive programs.

The first criticism concerns the inability of the available scientific data to prove conclusively that lowering individual risk factors will prevent or lessen the development of CHD. Although the vast bulk of experimental, clinical, and epidemiological evidence has consistently been able to associate certain risk factors with CHD, the crucial link proving that lessening individual risk factors will substantially lessen the risk of CHD is missing. Previous studies designed to substantiate this theory have been hampered by methodological flaws. Many studies, such as the Chicago Coronary Prevention and Evaluation Program, have reported decreased CHD morbidity and mortality in the control of multiple risk factors. The Multiple Risk Factor Intervention Trial (MRFIT) is a 6-year prospective clinical trial designed to demonstrate the effectiveness of primary prevention in decreasing CHD mortality [12]. Twelve thousand subjects between the ages of 35 and 57 years have been randomly divided into control and test groups. While the control groups receive their regular medical care, the test group receives a specific intervention program. Group techniques are used to motivate test patients to stop smoking, attain ideal body weight, and adopt a diet low in saturated fats. Preliminary results will be available within the next few years.

The second major criticism that has hampered the implementation of primary preventive programs for CHD is that relatively little is known about the potential hazards or undesirable consequences of such programs. Those who advocate caution cite such recent findings as the substitution of skim milk for whole milk in infants may impair normal central nervous system development. Similarly, little is known about the effects of other dietary changes.

There are those who believe that before preventive programs should be instituted, even more convincing evidence relating individual risk factors to the development of CHD and more information on the safety of preventive programs are necessary. There are those, however, who recognize that although there are limitations in the available scientific knowledge, the knowledge available is so persuasive and CHD is so rampant that the immediate application of preventive programs to lower risk factors is justified.

Life expectancy for white men between 40 and 70 years of age has changed very little from 1900 to 1970. The future life expectancy for a 40-year-old man in 1900 was 27.7 years, compared to 31.9 years in 1970. Similarly, the future life expectancy for a 70-year-old man in 1900 was 9.0 years, compared to 10.5 years in 1970. Recent figures, however, indicate a significantly decreased ischemic heart disease mortality rate. Between 1969 and 1975, there was a 15-percent reduction in ischemic heart disease mortality. The preventive potential for identifying and treating persons at high risk is significant. Assuming that the proportion of men with multiple risk factors could be halved and assuming that 20 percent of men could be shifted from very high risk status to a somewhat lower risk status, there would be approximately a 19-percent reduction in CHD mortality, saving approximately 45,000 lives per year.

PRIMARY PREVENTION

There is already some evidence that primary preventive programs are effective [1, 2]. Ever since the Surgeon General of the United States Public Health Service warned of the health hazards of tobacco consumption, particularly cigarette smoking, and ever since the American Heart Association recommended a decreased intake of saturated fats and cholesterol in the general American diet, there has been a decreasing mortality from CHD. Table 1-1 tabulates changes in life-style.

Although there is an association between a change in diet and decreasing mortality from CHD, the association is not necessarily causal. Other factors, such as exercise programs and better control of hypertension, may contribute to the

Preventive Primary Medicine

Table 1-1. Change in Per Capita Consumption in the United States, 1963–1976

Product	Change
All tobacco products	26.5% decline
Fluid milk and cream	20.5% decline
Butter	36.2% decline
Eggs	13.2% decline
Animal fats and oils	51.2% decline
Vegetable fats and oils	63.9% increase

Source: U.S. Department of Agriculture, *Agricultural Statistics,* Government Printing Office, Washington, D.C., 1976. Pp. 106, 142, 384, 414, 561.

decrease in CHD mortality. However, the fact that a significant change in eating habits occurs concomitantly with a decrease in vascular mortality is indeed impressive.

The Framingham Offspring Study provides additional indication that primary prevention may already be effective in decreasing CHD mortality [8]. In comparing the age-specific means of blood pressure, serum cholesterol, and cigarette smoking between the original cohorts and their offspring, there was a decrease in all three factors among the offspring. In men aged 30 to 39 years, for example, the mean systolic blood pressure decreased from 133 to 125 mm Hg (there was no change in diastolic readings). The mean serum cholesterol level decreased from 215 mg/100 ml to 200 mg/100 ml, and the percentage of smokers decreased from 70 to 45 percent. The observed decrease in CHD risk factors may be due to generally increased health awareness or to the institution of primary preventive measures.

No single risk factor is as effective in the detection of persons at high risk of developing CHD as are multiple risk factors [7]. Hypertension, hyperlipidemia, and smoking carry the greatest risk of a person's developing premature CHD. These conditions are easy to identify and amenable to therapy. Inactivity, obesity, and stress are also easy to identify but may be somewhat less amenable to therapy. These multiple risk factors are extremely common, and it has been estimated that up to 20 percent of a middle-aged population would fall into a high-risk group (Table 1-2).

To test the importance and utility of a coronary risk profile in identifying patients at risk of developing CHD, the coronary risk profiles of 158 patients undergoing cardiac catheterization and coronary angiography were compared [13, 19]. In this study, the risk profile was based on age, sex, cigarette smoking, glucose intolerance, systolic blood pressure, serum cholesterol, and electrocardiographic evidence of left ventricular hypertrophy. The principal finding was that the collection of routine clinical data can provide "penetrating insight" about the presence and severity of coronary artery disease. There was a steady progressive increase in the numbers and severity of coronary risk factors with each increment in severity of coronary artery disease. The higher-risk coronary patient can be identified on the basis of easily determined factors that correlate with the severity of angiographically determined coronary artery disease.

The overwhelming bulk of evidence already assembled makes clear that enough is known about the risk factors for CHD for the primary care physician to apply a rational program of primary prevention. The evidence for the causative role of diet, smoking, hypertension, and hyperlipidemia is beyond a reasonable doubt. The evidence for inactivity and psychological stress is weaker but very suggestive. Altering these risk factors may mean altering behavior and life-style. Although the primary care physician is in an optimum position to motivate and supervise many of these changes, changing lifetime patterns of middle-aged adults is difficult. Since the underlying, predisposing atherosclerotic process begins early in life, it is necessary to sow the seeds of prevention early in infancy and childhood. Prevention that begins early can be truly effective.

Table 1-2. *Percent Prevalance of Selected Risk Factors in the United States*

Age	Inactivity	Obesity	Hypertension	Smoking	Diabetes Mellitus	Hyper-cholesterolemia	ECG-LVH
Men							
35–44	12.1	12.5	13.5	48.6	1.1	20.2	2.9
45–54	16.9	14.7	18.3	43.1	1.1	25.7	4.8
55–64	21.0	12.5	27.3	37.4	3.3	23.5	10.0
65–74	27.1	12.7	27.1	27.8	3.2	21.6	7.1
Women							
35–44	13.3	20.1	8.5	38.8	0.8	12.9	0.9
45–54	19.3	24.2	18.2	36.1	2.9	28.0	3.6
55–64	30.8	30.9	31.2	24.2	3.2	49.7	4.1
65–74	39.0	27.2	47.6	10.2	6.1	51.0	9.6

ECG-LVH = electrocardiographic evidence of left ventricular hypertrophy.
Source: Kannel, McGee, and Gordon [14].

OBESITY

Prevention can begin with infant feeding practices. Breast-feeding should be encouraged, when possible, for the first few months of life. Bottle-feeding may be an important cause of obesity in infants. Unnecessary excess calories are often given. Cow's milk is higher in protein, saturated fats, and salt and lower in the essential fatty acids than breast milk. There is also some evidence that cow's protein may be antigenic to humans and may damage the arterial wall. The high salt content of infant foods may lead to excess thirst, which may in turn prompt the giving of milk instead of water, which may result in increased weight gain. Many babies are too fat and remain so throughout childhood and adult life.

Eating habits formed early in childhood are difficult to change later on. Poor eating habits may encourage obesity, high levels of blood lipids, and development of premature atherosclerosis. Obesity among children and adolescents is a considerable health problem in the United States. The Ten State Nutritional Survey, using triceps skin fold thickness to determine obesity, reported that among 12- and 13-year-olds, 17 percent of white boys, 12 percent of white girls, 9 percent of black boys, and 11 percent of black girls were obese. Overweight infants tend to become overweight children, who become overweight adults. In one study, 86 percent of overweight boys and 80 percent of overweight girls became overweight adults. The odds against an overweight adolescent becoming an average-weight adult are 28:1.

Obesity has already been implicated as a significant risk factor in hypertension and as a risk factor in CHD. In addition, obesity is associated with a variety of other physical problems, including decreased growth-hormone release, hyperinsulinemia, and carbohydrate intolerance. Psychologically, obese children show less acceptance by peers, have greater body-image disturbances, have poorer self-concepts, and show more evidence of disturbed personality characteristics than their normal-weight peers.

In view of the body of evidence implicating obesity as a risk factor in a variety of conditions, how can the primary care physician effectively prevent and, if necessary, treat obesity? Intervention begun early in life is crucial because young children can learn and utilize appropriate eating and exercise habits more easily than older children. Six basic approaches exist in treating obesity: (1) caloric restriction, (2) anorectic drugs, (3) physical exercise, (4) therapeutic starvation, (5) bypass surgery, and (6) habit-pattern changes based upon social learning theory [5].

The results of treating obese children have shown that clinically significant weight reduction occurred rarely. Following treatment, furthermore, obese children consistently failed to continue losing weight or to even maintain weight losses experienced during treatment.

The standard clinical practice of dietary counseling, usually at irregular intervals and for varying amounts of time, is not effective. In a sample of 269 obese schoolchildren seen in a clinic on a monthly basis for dietary counseling, none was able to achieve ideal weight and only 26 percent were able to decrease their weight to 25 percent above the appropriate weight. More encouraging results have been obtained with more intense and more frequent contact with patients. In a combination of inpatient and outpatient treatment, 10 out of 11 patients lost more than 10 pounds. Results of long-term follow-up, however, are still discouraging. Thus it is clear that dietary counseling by itself is generally ineffective in treating obesity in children. Intensive dietary counseling may be beneficial for short-term but not necessarily for long-term weight loss.

Anorectic drugs, which depress the appetite through stimulation of the central nervous system, generally have little effect in the treatment of obese children. The dropout rate is high. The short-term efficacy of the drugs is minimal, and follow-up data indicate complete relapse. Similarly, hormonal treatments have little beneficial effect.

Exercise programs do seem to have some value. In a study comparing exercise activity of obese and nonobese girls in a summer camp, it was clearly demonstrated that normal-weight adolescent girls were 2½ times more active than their overweight peers [5]. In a program combining nutritional education and daily exercise, there was an average 10.9-percent reduction in weight. However, for such programs to demonstrate lasting impact, evidence for continued weight loss and continued weight-loss maintenance is required.

Therapeutic starvation has been advocated for treating severely obese individuals. Benefits include a significant weight reduction within a short period of time and a predictable psychological boost for the patient. Recidivism, however, invariably occurs. Another popular variant of this technique is placing the individual in a special camp setting that controls the physical and social environment. These programs have been successful, but only for as long as the person remains within the controlled environment.

Bypass surgery is an extreme, last-ditch attempt to control weight in a grossly obese individual for whom all other methods have failed. Surgery has generally been limited to adults. Complications including diarrhea, vitamin B_{12} malabsorption, hypocalcemia, and fatty liver have all been reported.

Recently, several behavior modification programs have become increasingly popular. The behavioral approach alters food intake and exercise levels by modifying those variables believed to influence a person's food selection and activity patterns. Although behavior modification programs have brought new hope to the treatment of obesity in adults, few successes have been demonstrated in children. However, some of the characteristics of behavior modification programs, such as treating mothers and children together and emphasizing long-term involvement and gradual weight loss, may by themselves positively influence results.

In treating obesity, it is clear that interventions marked by a high degree of structure and supervision usually produce better short-term results. Family involvement is crucial to treatment success because obesity in both parents and children is positively correlated and because family support is important in influencing continued weight loss. Strategies designed to encourage, support, and teach beneficial eating and exercise habits outside of the regular treatment programs may positively influence treatment outcome. A successful treatment program must also include a follow-up program designed to decrease recidivism.

LOW-FAT DIETS

The association between diet and hyperlipidemia, atherosclerosis, and CHD is so impressive that the primary care physician has a responsibility to motivate and educate his patients to reduce the fat in their diets. The physician should strive for a modification of essential eating habits rather than for the avoidance of certain dishes. There is a far greater likelihood of successfully altering lifelong eating patterns if entire families become involved. Children will hopefully then learn good eating habits from their parents.

Specific dietary goals should aim toward adjusting the total caloric intake to achieve ideal body weight. Dietary cholesterol should be decreased to less than 300 mg per day from the 600 mg per day now present in the average American diet. Saturated fats should be decreased so that they constitute less than 10 percent of the total caloric intake.

If diet is to be effective in preventing atherosclerosis, lifelong changes in cooking and eating habits are necessary. Since eating is one of man's greatest pleasures, lifelong restrictions of fat intake through traditional "diets" that eliminate many pleasurable dishes are impractical. Instead, an attitude must be adopted of preparing and eating food that can offer the same variety of dishes and still restrict fat intake. The central theme of low-fat cooking is that by merely substituting low-fat items for high-fat items, the same variety of pleasurable dishes can be offered but with significantly reduced fat content. Through modifications in cooking technique, even further reductions are possible. For example, a cherry pie as usually cooked contains 93 gm of fat. By use of substitutions, the fat content can be decreased to 8 gm.

The current proliferation of new, low-fat food products makes low-fat cooking available to everyone. Better product labeling may also eventually aid the consumer in selecting low-fat foods. A detailed guide to low-fat cooking that includes low-fat recipes, instructions on lowering the visible and invisible fat content of food, and a list of the fat content of various foods, such as *Low-Fat Cookery* by Evelyn S. Stead and Gloria K. Warren (McGraw-Hill, New York, 1959), is invaluable.

HYPERLIPIDEMIA

Since the relationship between lipid levels and risk of CHD is continuous, reduction of hyperlipidemia is advantageous and should be pursued on a lifelong basis. Hyperlipidemia commonly occurs along with other risk factors such as hypertension and cigarette smoking, and many experts feel that the hyperlipidemia should not even be treated until the hypertension and cigarette smoking have been eliminated. Certainly, since risk factors seem to be additive, hyperlipidemic therapy should be part of a comprehensive program to reduce CHD risk factors. Table 1-3 lists the upper limits of the normal range for cholesterol and triglyceride concentrations in the blood according to age.

The most common cause of hypercholesterolemia is endogenous overproduction of cholesterol. Increased synthesis of cholesterol is also associated with obesity and hereditary factors. Familial hypercholesterolemia ac-

Table 1-3. *Age-related Upper Limits for*
Serum Cholesterol and Serum Triglyceride

Age	Serum Cholesterol (mg/100 ml)	Serum Triglyceride (mg/100 ml)
0–19	230	140
20–29	240	140
30–39	270	150
40–49	310	160
50–59	330	190

Source: Adapted from Jones [12].

counts for approximately 3 percent of premature coronary artery disease. The affected individual will have cholesterol levels as high as 350 to 450 mg/100 ml. Therapy for endogenous hypercholesterolemia is directed at decreasing cholesterol intake from the diet, decreasing hepatic synthesis through weight reduction, and increasing cholesterol catabolism to bile acid with the aid of drugs.

The most common cause of hypertriglyceridemia is excessive synthesis of hepatic triglyceride into the plasma. Endogenous triglyceride is synthesized from carbohydrate and fatty acid precursors. Triglyceride synthesis is stimulated by caloric excess, dietary carbohydrates, ethanol, estrogens, oral contraceptives, and states of hyperinsulinism such as may occur from obesity or corticosteroid excess.

Endogenous hypertriglyceridemia frequently is genetic. Treatment begins with a withdrawal of offending drugs such as estrogen, oral contraceptives, and corticosteroids. Diet therapy emphasizes caloric restriction in order to attain ideal body weight, alcohol restriction, and, if necessary, carbohydrate restriction. In addition, both nicotinic acid and clofibrate (Atromid-S) appear to decrease hepatic triglyceride synthesis.

Drug therapy for hyperlipidemia must be carefully selected, since the therapeutic regime must be followed for a lifetime to realize potential benefits. Clofibrate acts to decrease triglyceride concentrations by inhibiting hepatic triglyceride synthesis. Cholesterol synthesis also may be decreased. Clofibrate is a well-tolerated supplement to diet therapy in patients with hypertriglyceridemia. Potential side effects include dyspepsia, nausea, decreased libido, and impotence. Occasional allergic cutaneous reactions may occur. In the Coronary Drug Project, there was reported an increased incidence of thrombophlebitis, pulmonary embolism, and cardiac arrhythmias in patients taking clofibrate. It must also be pointed out that the rate of recurrent myocardial infarctions did not decrease in the 8 years of follow-up.

Nicotinic acid also decreases triglyceride synthesis and inhibits cholesterol synthesis. In the Coronary Drug Project, patients treated with nicotinic acid had a 29-percent reduction in nonfatal reinfarctions, as well as decreased evidence of angina pectoris. Common side effects, which usually disappear after 2 weeks of therapy, include cutaneous flushing and pruritus. Starting therapy with small doses of 100 mg, 3 times a day, and gradually increasing to 1 to 2 gm, 3 times a day, may reduce these effects. Other side effects, including gastric distress, dyspepsia, cutaneous hyperpigmentation, increased uric acid levels, and increased liver function tests, have also been reported.

Cholestyramine is the current drug of choice for treating isolated hypercholesterolemia. Unfortunately, patient acceptance of this drug is limited because of frequent gastrointestinal side effects. The drug is not absorbed and acts by binding bile salts, producing an increase in bioacid formation and a decrease in serum cholesterol. Constipation, bloating, nausea, and dyspepsia, although mild, are frequent side effects. Cholestyramine also inhibits absorption of fat-soluble vitamins and may decrease the half-life of drugs excreted by the bile such as digitalis and thyroxin.

PHYSICAL ACTIVITY

Since physical activity also seems to play an important role in decreasing CHD, the primary care physician should be prepared to structure and supervise a graduated exercise program for patients at risk. The President's Council on Physical Fitness and Sports obtained evaluations of 14 popular forms of exercise in terms of heart and lung endurance, muscular endurance, muscular strength, flexibility, balance, and general well-being (weight control, muscle definition, digestion, sleep). Each variable for each exercise was graded from zero to three by each of seven experts. The results are as follows:

Exercise	Total Rating
Jogging	147
Bicycling	142
Swimming	140
Skating	140
Handball, squash	140
Skiing—Nordic	139
Basketball	134
Skiing—Alpine	134
Tennis	128
Calisthenics	126
Walking	102
Golf (cart)	66
Softball	64
Bowling	51

The American Heart Association, the American College of Sports Medicine, and others agree that the most beneficial forms of exercise are the ones that contribute to cardiopulmonary conditioning. Many exercise programs, such as Dr. Cooper's Aerobics Program, the President's Guide of Physical Fitness, and the official YMCA exercise program, are excellent for this purpose. Since many of these programs may be demanding in terms of time and commitment, a flexible, individually tailored program

Table 1-4. *Target Heart Rate and Heart Rate Range*

Age	Maximum Heart Rate, Beats per Min.	Target Heart Rate (75% of Maximum), Beats per Min.	Heart Rate Range (70–85% of Maximum), Beats per Min.
20	200	150	140–170
25	195	146	137–166
30	190	142	133–162
35	185	139	130–157
40	180	135	126–153
45	175	131	123–149
50	170	127	119–145
55	165	124	116–140
60	160	120	112–136
65	155	116	109–132
70	150	112	105–128

Source: Consumer Guide [6].

based upon sound cardiopulmonary conditioning techniques may be more suitable. The Consumer Guide Program employs this approach for jogging [6]. Its principles may be transferred to other sports or forms of exercise.

Exercise contributes to cardiovascular conditioning only if it involves sustained action for at least 15 minutes at approximately 75 percent of the maximum heart rate. Maximum heart rate is generally calculated as 220 minus the individual's age. The target heart rate and heart rate range for various ages are listed in Table 1-4.

The basic principle of structuring an exercise program is to perform some exercise that will produce 75 percent of the individual's maximum heart rate for at least 15 minutes at least 3 times per week. Exercise below 75 percent of the maximum heart rate is insufficient for cardiopulmonary conditioning, while exercise above 75 percent of the maximum heart rate may be too strenuous. Naturally, a thorough physical evaluation is mandatory before recommending any exercise program, especially for individuals over age 35.

Summary and Recommendations

Diseases of the heart are the leading cause of death in the United States today. Because of the long natural history of atherosclerosis, late intervention can neither change the underlying pathological process nor contribute significantly to lowering the CHD death rate. Unlike late intervention, primary prevention can make significant contributions in controlling CHD. The primary care physician should consider all clinical cases of CHD as preventive medicine failures.

Diets high in saturated fats, hypercholesterolemia, hypertension, and cigarette smoking are major etiological risk factors for CHD. Obesity, sedentary living, psychosocial stress, glucose intolerance, and family history are secondary risk factors. Except for family history, all risk factors are amenable to change.

Up to 20 percent of a middle-aged population will be at great, some at very great, risk of developing clinical CHD. The primary care physician can accurately identify these patients by means of routine clinical information. Through education, motivation, and diligence, he must attempt to lower identified risk factors.

RECOMMENDATIONS

1. Diet—Diet forms a major weapon in the primary prevention of CHD.
   a. Breast-feeding of infants should be encouraged.
   b. Obesity in children should be discouraged.
   c. Families should be educated to alter their eating patterns in order to lower their fat intake to less than 300 mg of cholesterol per day.

d. All adults should be encouraged to reach and maintain ideal body weight.
2. Screening.
   a. Hypertension—Hypertension is a common condition even in childhood. All patients should have their blood pressure recorded during every visit to the physician. Adults should have their blood pressure checked at least every 2 years.
   b. Hypercholesterolemia—Hypercholesterolemia is associated with significant risk, and evidence indicates that treatment will reduce that risk. Screening of serum cholesterol should be done at least every 4 years. There is insufficient evidence to warrant screening for hypertriglyceridemia or typing of the hyperlipoproteinemia.
   c. Smoking—A smoking history should be obtained during the initial physical examination and should be repeated periodically, perhaps every 10 years.
   d. Obesity—The detection of obesity is simple. All adults should have height and weight measured at least every 4 years for comparison with tables of ideal body weights.
   e. Life-style—The primary care physician should be aware of the psychosocial stresses and exercise habits of his patients.

References

1. Ball, K., and R. Turner.   Realism in the prevention of coronary heart disease (editorial). *Prev. Med.* 4:390, 1975.
2. Borhani, N.   Opportunities for primary prevention of coronary heart disease. *Prev. Med.* 4:482, 1975.
3. Boyle, E.   Biological patterns of hypertension by race, sex, body weight, skin color. *J.A.M.A.* 213:1637, 1970.
4. Cantwell, J.   Running. *J.A.M.A.* 240:1409, 1978.
5. Coates, T., and C. Thoresen,   Treating obesity in children and adolescents: A review. *Am. J. Public Health* 68:143, 1978.
6. Consumer Guide (Eds).   *The Running Book.* Beekman House New York, 1978.
7. Cordraz, E., and S. Cordroy.   Prevention of heart disease by control of risk factors: The time has come to face the facts (editorial). *Am. J. Cardiol.* 35:330, 1975.
8. Feinleib, M., et al.   The Framingham Offspring Study: Design and preliminary data. *Prev. Med.* 4:518, 1975.
9. Genkins, D.   Recent evidence supporting psychological and social risk factors for coronary disease. *N. Engl. J. Med.* 294:987, 1976.

10. Gruskin, A. Clinical evaluation of hypertension in children. *Primary Care* 1:233, 1974.

11. Johnson, A. et al. Influences of race, sex and weight on blood pressure behavior in young adults. *Am. J. Cardiol.* 35:523, 1975.

12. Jones, R. The hyperlipoproteinemias: Detection, diagnosis and management. *Med. Clin. North Am.* 57:47, 1973.

13. Kannel, W. Some lessons in cardiovascular epidemiology from Framingham. *Am. J. Cardiol.* 37:269, 1976.

14. Kannel, W., D. McGee, and T. Gordon. A general cardiovascular risk profile: The Framingham Study. *Am. J. Cardiol.* 38:46, 1976.

15. Klatsky, A., Friedman, C., and Siegelaub, A. Alcohol consumption on blood pressure: Kaiser-Permanente multiphasic health examination data. *N. Engl. J. Med.* 296:1194, 1977.

16. Multiple risk factor intervention trial: A national study of primary prevention of coronary heart disease (review). *J.A.M.A.* 235:825, 1976.

17. Reisin, E., et al. Effect of weight loss without salt restriction on the reduction of blood pressure in overweight hypertensive patients. *N.Engl. J. Med.* 298:1, 1978.

18. Report of the Inter Society Commission for Heart Disease Resources. Primary prevention of atherosclerotic diseases. *Circulation* 42:55, 1970.

19. Salel, A., et al. Accuracy of numerical coronary profile. *N. Engl. J. Med.* 296:1447, 1977.

20. Stamler, J. Epidemiology of coronary heart disease. *Med. Clin. North Am.* 57:5, 1973.

21. Turner, R., and K. Ball. The cardiologist's responsibility for preventing coronary heart disease. *Am. Heart J.* 91:139, 1976.

22. Walker, W. Changing U.S. life style and declining vascular mortality: Cause or coincidence? *N. Engl. J. Med.* 297:163, 1977.

2

Cerebrovascular Disease

Occurrence

Cerebrovascular disease is the third leading cause of death in the United States, accounting for two hundred thousand deaths annually. In 1975, it constituted 10.2 percent of all deaths. Although stroke is usually considered a disease of old age, two-thirds of all strokes and almost one-fifth of all stroke deaths occur in persons under age 65. A community study, which can avoid many of the sampling biases of hospital, autopsy, or mortality series, has shown high prevalence rates of cerebral symptoms. Of 2,455 persons over age 40 sampled, 15.9 per 1,000 white men, 11.5 per 1,000 white women, 7.0 per 1,000 black men, and 7.8 per 1,000 black women had existing or prior cerebral symptoms [15]. Between 1950 and 1975, the overall death rate from cerebrovascular disease dropped 41 percent (Fig. 2-1). This significant decrease is mostly due to a decline in mortality for those under age 50. For those over age 50, the death rate has not changed significantly in the past 25 years.

Etiology

Data from the Framingham Study, in which 5,106 persons aged 30 to 62 were followed continuously, reveal the

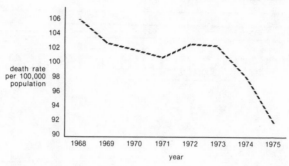

Figure 2-1. *Death rate by year from cerebrovascular disease.*

causes and average age of strokes listed in Table 2-1 [14].
Strokes in persons under 50 years of age are most often
due to embolism or to subarachnoid hemorrhage secondary to embolism. Embolic processes secondary to rheumatic heart disease, myocardial infarction with mural
thrombi, and subacute bacterial endocarditis are common
sources. Less common nonatherosclerotic causes of stroke
in those under age 50 are vasculitides caused either by a
specific agent such as tuberculosis or syphilis or by unknown agents such as systemic lupus erythematosus
(where there is a 75-percent incidence of neurological involvement) and hematological disorders associated with
intravascular coagulation [16]. The decline in stroke
mortality for those under age 50 may be attributed to improvement in the treatment of the underlying diseases
causing embolic phenomena.

In the older population, atherosclerosis is the major
cause of stroke. The death rate from atherosclerotic-related
strokes has not improved as it has in nonatherosclerotic
strokes.

Cerebrovascular atherosclerosis is part of a larger, more
widespread pathophysiological process of atherosclerosis.
Major risk factors leading to the development of atherosclerosis are increased blood pressure, a diet high in satu-

Table 2-1. *Relative Frequency of Cerebrovascular Lesions*

Type of Lesion	Percentage	Patient Age
Thrombosis	63	59 yr
Subarachnoid hemorrhage	18	56 yr
Embolus	15	50 yr
Intracerebral hemorrhage	4	62 yr

Source: Adapted from Kannel et al. [14].

rated fats and cholesterol, and cigarette smoking. There is somewhat less convincing evidence to implicate obesity, hyperglycemia, and sedentary living. The role of psychosocial tension in the etiology of atherosclerosis is not yet clear [13]. Identification and reduction of any of the risk factors relating to atherosclerosis can in turn decrease stroke morbidity and mortality.

Because preventive measures directed at reducing atherosclerosis will have a large impact on decreasing stroke morbidity and mortality, the primary care physician must be responsible for assessing and lowering, if possible, those risk factors associated with the atherosclerotic process. Although the present understanding of the causal mechanisms leading to the development of atherosclerosis precludes dogmatism, detection and control of hypertension are essential. Encouraging a diet low in saturated fats seems reasonable and desirable. Elimination of smoking, maintenance of ideal body weight, and moderate exercise may also retard the atherosclerotic process [13].

Until a safe and effective approach to the prevention of the atherosclerotic process is found, the prevention of stroke can be improved by (1) identifying and treating stroke risk factors, (2) recognizing and treating transient ischemic attacks, and (3) recognizing and appropriately treating neck murmurs.

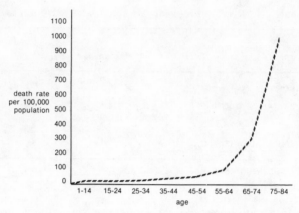

Figure 2-2. *Death rate by age from cerebrovascular disease, 1975.*

Risk Factors

AGE

The incidence of stroke increases with age. The death rate rises from 12 deaths per 100,000 at age 30 to 91 deaths per 100,000 at age 60 to 1,096 deaths per 100,000 at age 80 (Fig. 2-2).

CARDIAC DISEASE

In the Framingham Study, the risk of stroke was five times greater for persons with coronary heart disease than for those without it. Persons with electrocardiographic evidence of left ventricular hypertrophy (LVH) have nine times the risk of stroke than those without such evidence of LVH [14].

HYPERTENSION

Hypertensives have more strokes than normotensives. Data from several prospective studies have shown that hypertension is the most potent known predicting factor for stroke. Although no critical level of blood pressure exists, the morbidity ratio increases with each higher level of blood pressure. If blood pressure exceeds 160 mm Hg systolic or 95 mm Hg diastolic, the risk of stroke is four times greater than for normotensives [17].

Despite the central importance of blood pressure control in decreasing the incidence of stroke, it has been estimated that only 9 percent of all hypertensives under treatment are in good control. In a household survey, 42 percent of hypertensives found did not even know that they were hypertensive. Less than one-third who knew they were hypertensive were being treated [19].

As a result of this poor record, significant efforts, both private and governmental, have been made to identify and bring adequate treatment to the millions of Americans believed to have high blood pressure. Systematic educational campaigns and screening programs have had a substantial impact. A recent survey of employed persons showed that 86 percent found to have high blood pressure were aware of their condition, compared to only 57 percent 10 years earlier [1]. In addition, 66 percent of those hypertensives indicated that they were receiving some treatment for their high blood pressure, compared to only 36 percent receiving treatment 10 years earlier.

Although a greater proportion of people have become aware of their condition and a greater proportion have received some type of treatment, unfortunately the percentage of those adequately treated has remained constant. In a 1960–1962 survey, 50 percent of those receiving treatment for hypertension were adequately treated. In a 1970–1972 survey, 50 percent also were adequately treated [1].

This situation exists despite the availability of effective therapy, which, if applied, could dramatically decrease the incidence of vascular disease. Clearly, if the potential of effective chemotherapy of hypertension is to be realized, methods for care must be improved.

In one study of high blood pressure at a university general medical clinic, the treatment of hypertension was found to be unsatisfactory for most patients [1]. One-half of all hypertensive patients were lost to follow-up within the first year. Satisfactory control was achieved by only one-third of the patients. This study clearly demonstrates that the university general medical clinic is doing a relatively poor job of hypertension control. Since up to 20 percent of all ambulatory care is provided by hospital clinics, serious consideration should be given to providing alternative methods of control for uncomplicated hypertension.

Better results have been obtained with programs specifically designed to serve patients with moderate uncomplicated hypertension. A common characteristic of such programs is facilitated access to a system of medical care where paraprofessionals administer care under a standard protocol. Such programs emphasize health education and self-care and provide an environment of concern and understanding for chronic illness.

One such program used the work site to detect and treat hypertension [2]. In this program all care was provided at the work site. An introductory educational campaign was followed by blood pressure screening of employees. Those employees with blood pressure greater than 160/95 mm Hg were invited for two confirmation tests at weekly intervals. Eligible employees were seen by a nurse, who obtained a preliminary history and laboratory data. One week later, a physician obtained a history, performed a physical examination, and reviewed the laboratory data. The initial therapy was begun with hydrochlorothiazide. Subsequent treatment followed a specific protocol. A nurse saw patients at weekly intervals and then at decreasing intervals as blood pressure control was achieved. During these visits, besides monitoring blood pressure control, therapy, and complications, the nurse sought to increase patient understanding and involvement.

In this program, 84 percent of employees were screened. Sixty-five percent of those with confirmed hypertension elected to participate in the program. An impressive 97 percent of these patients remained in therapy after 1 year, and an equally impressive 81 percent had satisfactory blood pressure reduction. Although these figures suggest that a program linking detection to treatment in an accessible setting where patient education is central can be very successful, other studies indicate that labeling patients as hypertensive resulted in increased absenteeism from work [12]. In one study, absenteeism among workers screened and referred for hypertension increased 71 percent over the general employee population. The main factor associated with this increased absenteeism was the employees' becoming aware of their hypertension.

Labeling persons as hypertensive should therefore only be done after the diagnosis has been firmly established by serial blood pressure measurements. Further, detection should only be carried out in settings in which proper treatment and follow-up care can be assured.

Although the primary care physician may not run community-based hypertension control programs, he is in an ideal position to adopt some of the key elements from these programs that have proved successful. The primary care physician can facilitate access to care, he can link detection with treatment, and he can provide an environment conducive to long-term patient compliance. He may want to adhere to a protocol of care and may want to use paraprofessionals, under his supervision, for continual surveillance and patient education.

In any event, the advent of a large array of effective medications, coupled with the knowledge that treatment of patients with established hypertension is beneficial, has provided the primary care physician with the necessary incentive and tools to treat hypertension.

Treatment of hypertension is a major example of effective preventive medicine. Young hypertensive patients are at increased risk for developing heart disease, stroke, and renal failure. It is this young population, especially those without any objective signs of cardiovascular damage, who stand to gain the most from early treatment.

As a rule, unless the blood pressure is very high or there are objective vascular complications, the decision to start treatment should be based upon more than one casual reading. Usually three successive readings at weekly intervals are adequate to make a judgment. In addition to the actual level of blood pressure, such factors as sex and race may contribute to the decision. Men, generally, are at greater risk than women for hypertensive complications and probably should be treated at an earlier stage. Blacks are more susceptible than whites to complications and should receive more aggressive therapy.

Objective signs of vascular damage provide additional incentives to start treatment, even when blood pressure levels are only minimally elevated. Changes in the optic fundi, electrocardiographic evidence of LVH or ischemia, and biochemical evidence of decreased renal function present strong indications for treatment.

Other risk factors for hypertension such as family history of hypertension or cardiovascular disease may tilt the scales toward early treatment. Concomitant risk factors such as obesity, diabetes mellitus, and hyperlipidemia commonly occur among hypertensives and need to be treated as well.

In addition to specific antihypertensive chemotherapy, several nonspecific approaches can be beneficial. Diet may play an important role, especially for those hypertensive patients who are obese. Recent evidence shows that a reduction in weight generally results in a reduction in blood pressure. Sodium retention plays a role in sustaining increased blood pressure among some patients. To produce volume depletion equivalent to that of a mild diuretic, however, requires a strict and therefore unpalatable diet. A reasonable compromise is to recommend a no-added-salt diet, which can effectively decrease the sodium content from the average 12 gm to 4 gm of sodium per day.

Recent studies have shown that regular intake of excessive amounts of alcohol exacerbates hypertension. While reasonable amounts of alcohol probably have no deleterious effects, hypertensive patients should be advised to be prudent in their consumption of alcohol.

The role of exercise in hypertension is not clearly defined. Exercise does promote general cardiovascular fitness, however, and therefore a moderate degree of regular exercise is potentially beneficial.

Specific antihypertensive chemotherapy generally follows a stepped care approach that employs an additive sequence of medication. The protocol begins with a diuretic. Most hypertension can be controlled with diuretics alone. For those patients whose hypertension cannot be adequately controlled by diuretics, additional drugs are prescribed until satisfactory control is achieved.

The stepped care system using a diuretic as the cornerstone of therapy is rational if hypertension is due primarily to salt and water retention. Recent evidence seems to indicate, however, that the renin-angiotensin-aldosterone axis plays a major role in blood pressure control [18]. Recent progress in renin profiling has made it possible to distinguish high, medium, and low renin producers. Hypertension may be dependent upon an abnormality of renin production that inappropriately produces vasoconstriction.

When renin levels were measured in a group of essential hypertensives, 15 percent were found to be high renin producers, 55 percent were medium producers, and 30 percent were low producers. When studied epidemiologically, the high-renin group had higher diastolic values and a higher incidence of proteinuria, retinopathy, and hypokalemia. Since the high-renin patients were younger, it is likely that these patients are at greater risk for vascular complications. Indeed, 14 percent of the high-renin group had strokes, compared to 10 percent of the normals and none in the low-renin group. These figures make it seem rational to address the renin factor directly in therapy.

It now seems that essential hypertension, rather than being considered a uniform disease, should be considered a group of disorders caused by different biochemical mechanisms. If the role of renin is indeed essential, high-renin patients should be treated with antirenin therapy, while low-renin patients should continue to be treated with antivolume therapy. Medium-renin patients may require a combination of both antirenin and antivolume therapy.

In contrast to the traditional treatment protocol that starts with a diuretic, an alternative system first employs antirenin therapy on the assumption that high-renin producers are at greater risk for vascular complications. Although a wide variety of antivolume diuretics are available, the major specific antirenin drugs are the beta adrenergic blockers. Other antihypertensive agents, particularly clonidine, have some antirenin effect. Propranolol, the major beta blocker, depresses renin through direct action on the juxtaglomerular cells. Propranolol, unless contraindicated, is generally well tolerated and has a minimun of side effects. It does not produce postural changes and only rarely interferes with sexual potency.

In the absence of specific renin profiling, this approach recommends that all patients, exccept where contraindicated, be started on antirenin therapy. Propranolol is most often used in an average starting dose of 40 to 80 mg twice a day. If the starting dose succeeds in normalizing blood pressure, it can be gradually reduced to test for the lowest effective maintenance dose. If it is not completely effective, the dose can be increased to up to 320 mg per day. If complete correction is still not achieved, a diuretic can be added to treat volume factors. Up to 85 percent of hypertensive patients can be controlled with this regime. After normalization, the propranolol is gradually subtracted to see if the patient can be maintained on a diuretic alone.

For those comparatively few patients who cannot be controlled by this approach, other drugs can be empirically added.

CHOLESTEROL

Data from the Framingham Study showed a correlation between thromboembolic strokes and cholesterol level [14]. Another study found that the association between hyperlipidemia and increased stroke was limited to those under 50 years old. But for this age group hyperlipidemia represented a tenfold excess risk for stroke. Another study showed that persons with cholesterol levels over 250 mg/100 ml had three times the risk of stroke as persons with cholesterol levels under 190 mg/100 ml. The Wadsworth VA Clinical Diet Study showed the increased sensitivity of strokes to diet. Compared to matched controls on a normal diet, subjects receiving a diet high in unsaturated fats had a 41-percent lower stroke rate [17].

SMOKING

The Framingham Study demonstrated a linear association between cigarette smoking and incidence of stroke [14]. The greater the number of cigarettes smoked, the higher the incidence of stroke. Persons smoking one pack per day have five times the risk of stroke as nonsmokers [17].

TRANSIENT ISCHEMIC ATTACKS

Transient ischemic attacks (TIAs) are episodes of focal neurological deficit that return to normal status within 24 hours. Just as angina may portend infarction, TIAs may portend completed stroke. Symptoms of transient cerebral ischemia may be classified into those referrable to the carotid vessels and those referrable to the vertebrobasilar vessels. It has been estimated that one-third of all strokes are caused by lesions in the extracranial carotid circulation [10]. Carotid lesions in the neck are most common and generally involve the carotid bifurcation and the first 1 or

2 cm of the internal carotid artery. Microemboli origi-
nating in lesions at this site break off and are carried to
the intracerebral circulation, most commonly the middle
cerebral artery. They may also enter the ophthalmic artery
and less commonly the anterior and posterior cerebral
arteries. Hemiparesis, hemianesthesia, headache, and dys-
phagia, which may occur singularly or in combination, are
the most common symptoms.

Symptom	*Incidence*
Hemianesthesia	33%
Hemiparesis	31%
Headache	25%
Dysphagia	20%
Visual field disturbance	14%
Monoparesis	7%
Confusion	5%
Facial paresthesias	4%
Dysarthria	3%

The vertebrobasilar arteries are also commonly the site
of severe atherosclerosis. Vertigo is the most common
symptom of vertebrobasilar insufficiency. Visual field disturbances, drop attacks, and sensory disturbances of the
face may suggest vertebrobasilar TIAs.

Since most patients with TIAs undergo some form of
treatment, it is difficult to gather information on the natural history of TIAs. One author reports that there is a tendency for TIAs to cease spontaneously after 1 to 3 years
in at least 50 percent of cases [6]. Recent studies indicate
that patients with TIAs subsequently experience stroke in
22 to 36 percent of cases. In a prospective analysis of 79
patients with TIAs, 37 percent had new cerebrovascular
events. In this study, patients with multiple, repeated TIAs
had more new episodes than patients who had had only a
single episode.

The interval from the onset of a TIA to the development
of a completed stroke is much shorter for patients with

carotid insufficiency than for patients with vertebrobasilar insufficiency. In one group of 68 stroke patients, those with carotid insufficiency averaged a 14-month interval between the onset of the TIA and development of the stroke, compared to a 23-month interval for those with vertebrobasilar insufficiency. Another study emphasized the risk during the period immediately following an episode of carotid insufficiency. Of those that developed a stroke (37%), one-half occurred during the first year and one-fifth occurred during the first month after the first attack [19].

Medical Therapy. Since up to 36 percent of patients with TIAs will develop a completed stroke, proper management of the TIA is important. There is little evidence that once the atherosclerotic process becomes clinically manifest medical therapy can reverse it. Although anticoagulation can decrease the frequency of TIAs, there is conflicting evidence as to whether anticoagulation can also prevent subsequent stroke. Three large studies have suggested that anticoagulation treatment has helped prevent stroke in patients with TIAs. Two large studies have suggested that it did not [3]. Randomized trials of anticoagulation in patients with TIAs show a decreased frequency of TIAs and a small decrease in the incidence of completed stroke and stroke-related death in the anticoagulation group [6]. However, since the major cause of death among patients with stroke is cardiovascular disease in the form of myocardial infarction, there is little difference in mortality between treatment and nontreatment groups.

Long-term anticoagulation therapy poses significant risks and difficulties. To decrease the complications of long-term therapy, it is generally recommended that an anticoagulant be given for 3 to 6 months and then discontinued. A recent study suggests that the most beneficial effect of anticoagulation occurs within 2 months after the onset of the first TIA.

Newer drugs, particularly the nonsteroidal anti-inflammatory agents, such as dipyridamole and aspirin, have been able to decrease thrombus formation in artificially damaged arteries of experimental animals. The therapeutic role for these antiplatelet aggregating drugs is unclear. Large cooperative studies are now in progress to evaluate their effectiveness in decreasing the initial stages of intra-arterial thrombosis.

In the Canadian Cooperative Study, 585 patients with threatened stroke were followed in a randomized clinical trial for 26 months to determine whether aspirin with sulfinpyrazone influenced the subsequent occurrence of TIAs, stroke, or death [5]. Aspirin significantly reduced the risk of continued TIAs, stroke, and death. Among men, there was up to a 48-percent reduction in risk for stroke or death. There was no significant reduction among women. According to this carefully controlled study, aspirin in the dose of 300 mg, 4 times per day, should be prescribed, unless contraindicated, to substantially decrease the risk of stroke among men experiencing TIAs.

Surgical Therapy. Surgery is a useful preventive measure against stroke for patients with extracranial carotid artery occlusive disease. Vertebrobasilar occlusive disease is not ordinarily amenable to surgical correction. The principal role of surgery in the management of patients with carotid artery occlusive disease is to remove arterial lesions that are potential sources of cerebral ischemia. Several large prospective and retrospective studies have determined the risks and long-term benefits of surgery. Other studies have determined the risks of the prerequisite diagnostic tests and the indications and contraindications for surgery. Only a minority of patients are surgical candidates. Patients with acute stroke and stroke in evolution are usually not considered surgical candidates. Criteria for remedial arterial surgery include the following [4]:

1. Clinical evaluation reveals the patient can tolerate major surgery.

2. History of TIAs.
3. If stroke has occurred, there is little neurological deficit.
4. At least 50-percent stenosis in one carotid artery.
5. If both carotids are stenotic, the symptomatic side must have at least 30-percent occlusion.
6. An ulcerated carotid plaque.
7. If more than one stenotic lesion is present, the accessible proximal one must be more stenotic.

Angiography is the definitive diagnostic test that must be performed prior to endarterectomy. Although generally considered "safe," it is not without significant morbidity, mortality, and discomfort. Several large studies have evaluated the complication rate of angiography [8]. A 1965 series of 1,703 patients reported permanent complications in 2.0 percent of patients. A 1968 series of 4,748 patients showed serious complications in 1.2 percent of patients and minor complications in 5.3 percent. A 1973 study of 2,000 patients found an average complication rate of 2.25 percent with death occurring in 0.1 percent, permanent neurological deficit in 0.25 percent, and transient neurological complications in 1.25 percent of cases.

Reports of surgical mortality from endarterectomy have been steadily decreasing. In 1965, mortality averaged 5 percent. This rate has decreased to an average of 1- to 2-percent mortality in 1975 [11].

Both medical and surgical therapy can decrease the frequency of TIAs. There is evidence that the risk of future stroke is less after surgery than after medical therapy. However, this decreased risk must be balanced against the increased mortality in the surgical group. A further benefit of surgery is that the complications of long-term anticoagulation are eliminated. A series of 316 patients with TIAs were randomized into medical and surgical treatment groups to determine the relative benefits of medical versus surgical treatment [10]. In the surgical group, surgical mortality was 1.6 percent, and the postoperative stroke rate was 4.8 percent. Subsequent TIAs occurred in 38 percent of the surgical group versus 54 percent of the medical group. New strokes occurred in 4 percent of the surgical group versus 12.4 percent of the medical group.

CAROTID BRUITS

Since a neck bruit may indicate roughening of the intima of the underlying artery, neck auscultation is a valuable indicator of extracranial arterial lesions. The coexistence of bruits over the carotid artery in the neck and extracranial carotid artery occlusive disease has been known for years. A bruit may exist without denoting stenosis, just as a bruit may not be audible in patients experiencing transient strokes who have significant stenosis. To document the specificity of neck auscultation, angiographic findings were compared with the auscultatory findings of 417 patients [7]. In asymptomatic patients, 65 percent of carotid arteries with bruits were associated with stenotic lesions. In patients with TIAs, 75 percent of carotid arteries with bruits were associated with stenotic lesions. Since from one-fourth to one-third of bruits heard were not associated with angiographically demonstrated stenosis, false positive findings are common. It was found that the presence of a bruit is often not as important as its location, quality, and intensity. Internal carotid artery stenosis most often causes loud and harsh bruits usually heard high in the neck just below the angle of the jaw.

The management of an asymptomatic carotid bruit is controversial [9]. Although there is no statistical data to support the benefit of elective surgery, some clinicians recommend angiography. Others suggest frequent observation. If the bruit changes, usually to a higher frequency indicating increased stenosis, then angiography and possible corrective surgery are recommended. An alternative approach is to monitor patients with asymptomatic carotid bruits with serial ophthalmodynamometry [11].

Summary and Recommendations

Cerebrovascular disease is the third leading cause of death in the United States. The reduction in overall stroke mortality in the last 25 years reflects an improvement in the treatment of the 15 percent of strokes caused by embolic diseases in those under age 50. For the almost two-thirds of strokes caused by atherosclerosis, there has been little decrease in mortality.

Identifying and lowering the risk factors associated with the atherosclerotic process will have a significant impact on lowering stroke mortality. Until an effective cure for atherosclerosis is found, control of hypertension, associated cardiac disease, and hypercholesterolemia and elimination of smoking will reduce stroke mortality.

Up to 37 percent of patients with transient ischemic attacks will develop strokes, many within 1 month of the first attack. Medical therapy can reduce the frequency of TIAs, but this therapy may not prevent subsequent strokes. Surgical therapy is a proven preventive measure for stroke in selected cases of extracranial carotid occlusive disease.

Carotid bruits may indicate extracranial occlusive disease. The location, intensity, and quality of the bruit are important in identifying significant neck bruits.

RECOMMENDATIONS

1. Stroke risk factors should be identified and treated.
2. Transient ischemic attacks should be identified and treated.
3. Neck bruits should be identified and appropriately treated.

References

1. Alderman, M., and O. Ochs. Treatment of hypertension at the university medical clinic, *Arch. Intern. Med.* 137:1707, 1977.
2. Alderman, M., and E. Schoenbaum. Detection and treatment of hypertension at the work site. *N. Engl. J. Med.* 293:65, 1975.

3. Browder, A., and J. Browder. Prevention of strokes. *Postgrad. Med.* 57:91, 1975.
4. Brown, D. Extracranial carotid atherosclerosis. *J. Ky. Med. Assoc.* 74:167, 1976.
5. Canadian Cooperative Study Group. A randomized trial of aspirin and sulfinpyrazone in threatened stroke. *N. Engl. J. Med.* 299:53, 1978.
6. Caronna, J. Transient ischemic attacks. *Postgrad. Med.* 59: 106, 1976.
7. David, T., et al. A correlation of neck bruits and arteriosclerotic carotid arteries. *Arch. Surg.* 107:729, 1973.
8. Deck, M. Radiologic examination of patients with stroke. *Postgrad. Med.* 59:123, 1976.
9. Fields, D.S., et al. Joint study of extracranial arterial occlusion. *J.A.M.A.* 211:1993, 1970.
10. Fields, D.S., and N. Lemak. Joint study of extracranial arterial occlusion. *J.A.M.A.* 235:2608, 1976.
11. Fraser, R. The role of surgery in ischemic stroke. *Postgrad. Med.* 59:135, 1976.
12. Haynes, R., et al. Increased absenteeism from work after detection and labeling of hypertensive patients. *N. Engl. J. Med.* 299:741, 1978.
13. Inter Society Commission for Heart Disease Resources. Primary prevention of atherosclerotic diseases. *Circulation* 42:55, 1970.
14. Kannel, W.B., et al. Vascular disease of the brain: Epidemiological aspects—The Framingham Study. *Am. J. Public Health* 55:1355, 1965.
15. Karp, H., et al. Transient cerebral ischemia: Prevalence and prognosis in a bi-racial rural community. *J.A.M.A.* 225:125, 1973.
16. Levine, J., and P. Swanson. Non atherosclerotic causes of stroke. *Ann. Intern. Med.* 70:807, 1969.
17. Walker, W. Success story: The program against major coronary risk factors. *Geriatrics* 31:97, 1976.
18. Weber, M., and J. Laragh. Hypertension. In H.F. Conn (Ed.), *Current Therapy, 1978.* Saunders, Philadelphia, 1978. Pp. 206–223.
19. Whismont, J. Epidemiology of stroke: Emphasis on transient cerebral ischemic attacks and hypertension. *Stroke* 5:68, 1974.

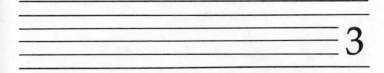

Cancer of the Lung

Occurrence

Cancer of the lung is the leading cause of male cancer death and the fourth leading cause of female cancer death in the United States. Incidence and mortality are increasing yearly, making lung cancer a growing public health problem. Before 1930, the death rates from lung cancer for both sexes were low and approximately equal. Since the 1930s, there has been a striking and rapid increase in male mortality (Fig. 3-1). Although female mortality has increased at a slower rate, there has been a recent marked increase in the death rate for women. The overall incidence of 3 deaths per 100,000 in 1930 rose to 34 deaths per 100,000 in 1970 to 42 deaths per 100,000 in 1975. Despite the rapid and continuing rise in incidence, the 5-year survival rate for bronchogenic carcinoma has remained constant at 5 to 10 percent. Since cigarette smoking is the major factor in the causation of lung cancer, most lung cancer is potentially preventable.

Etiology and Risk Factors

SMOKING

The carcinogenic potential of cigarette smoke is well estab-

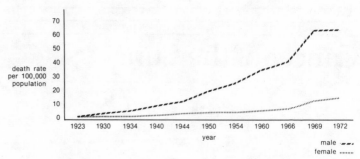

Figure 3-1. Death rate by year from lung cancer.

lished and is based upon the following types of evidence [12] :

1. At least 27 separate retrospective studies have demonstrated that the risk of lung cancer increases with the number of cigarettes smoked. Several large prospective studies have also confirmed this relationship.
2. The incidence of lung cancer is correlated with smoking habits. For example, lung cancer is rare among nonsmoking populations, such as Seventh Day Adventists. The increase in male and female lung cancer rates reflects the increase in male and female smoking habits.
3. Among ex-smokers, the rate of lung cancer declines, depending on the duration and the amount the person has smoked. The death rate from lung cancer among British physicians (who gave up cigarette smoking to a greater extent than the general population) decreased by 38 percent over a 10-year period. The risk of developing lung cancer after not smoking for 10 years declines to that of nonsmokers. The death rate from lung cancer among ex-smokers 50 to 69 years old who smoked 20 or more cigarettes per day declined to that of nonsmokers 10 years after giving up smoking.
4. In the experimental setting, tobacco tar has produced cancer in animals.

Ever since the distribution of the 1964 Surgeon General's Report, it is less and less disputed that tobacco smoking is causally related to lung cancer. Several variables, however, can modify the risk of developing lung cancer.

1. Amount smoked—The more an individual smokes, the greater his chances of developing cancer. The average male cigarette smoker has approximately ten times the risk of developing lung cancer compared to nonsmokers. Heavy smokers have at least twenty times the risk.
2. Smoking intensity factors—Such factors as duration of smoking, age on onset, and inhaling affect the risk of developing lung cancer [1].
3. Cigarette factors—The lower the content of tobacco tar, the lower the risk of developing lung cancer. There is also some evidence of decreased risk for filter users. Filter smokers need to smoke more cigarettes to have the same risk as nonfilter smokers [6].

OCCUPATIONAL EXPOSURE

It is well known that workers exposed to uranium, asbestos, chromate, nickel, and arsenic have an increased risk of developing lung cancer. On the average, the risk of developing lung cancer for workers exposed to these materials is four to eight times that of the general population, with higher rates prevailing among subgroups of workers exposed to hazardous processes [5].

Although the risk of occupational exposure is known, it was, until recently, believed to be confined to the workplace. Recent evidence has suggested that the risk may not be confined to the workplace at all but may be spread throughout the surrounding community. The first hint of widespread hazards of industrial processes came from asbestos studies [10]. Mortality studies had already demonstrated that asbestos-factory workers, even those with low exposure, had an increased risk of developing lung cancer. The effect of asbestos outside the workplace was first suspected when the presence of asbestos bodies among the general population was demonstrated. Although at present there is no known increased risk to the community resulting from low-level asbestos exposure, the spread of industrial hazards to the community is potentially alarming. Two subsequent studies on the geographical patterns of lung cancer document the community's risk of industrial hazards.

Previous studies had already shown that smelter workers exposed to high levels of arsenic emitted as a by-product of copper, lead, zinc, gold, and silver processing had a three- to eightfold excess risk of developing lung cancer. In a study of lung cancer mortalities in counties surrounding lead, copper, and zinc industries, there was a 17-percent excess increase among men and a 15-percent excess increase among women in lung cancer mortality [4]. A more recent survey of mortality by county in the United States reveals an excess mortality in counties where paper, chemicals, petroleum, and transportation industries are located. The elevated mortality occurred in the Northeast, around large metropolitan areas, and in a series of counties along the Gulf of Mexico and the Southeast Atlantic coast. The clustering of increased mortality suggests that environmental and industrial factors other than smoking may have a sizeable influence upon lung cancer risk [5].

AIR POLLUTION

Urban dwellers are estimated to have two times the incidence of pulmonary cancer as their rural counterparts. Although no specific air pollutant has been proved to cause lung cancer in humans, polycyclic organic matter has been implicated because similar compounds are present in cigarette smoke. Benzo[a]pyrene has been used as an index of urban pollution, and it is estimated that an increase in urban pollution as measured by benzo[a]pyrene levels corresponds with an increase in lung cancer deaths [1].

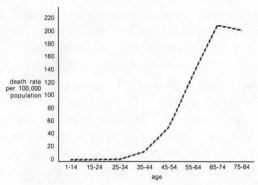

Figure 3-2. *Death rate by age from lung cancer, 1975.*

AGE

There is a correlation between age and incidence of lung cancer. Lung cancer is uncommon in persons under 45 years old. The death rate for 30-year-olds is 1 death per 100,000, which rises to 53 deaths per 100,000 by age 50 and to 211 deaths per 100,000 by age 70 (Fig. 3-2).

SEX

Men have a four-times greater risk of developing lung cancer than women. The annual male death rate is 60.3 deaths per 100,000, compared to an annual female death rate of 14.8 deaths per 100,000.

Screening

There is general agreement that mass screening for lung cancer is impractical. Screening should be confined to high-risk groups. The survival rate of persons with bronchogenic carcinoma will improve if tumors can be detected while still resectable. As long as surgery remains the best treatment, efforts to establish early diagnosis through effective screening programs must continue. In contrast to the progress made in the early detection of other cancers, until recently, little progress has been made in the recognition of early lung cancer. Chest x-ray and sputum cytology remain the only accepted screening tests. Although they are not ideal screening procedures, a screening program combining frequent chest x-rays and sputum cytologies can improve early detection. The major hope, however, for decreasing lung cancer mortality lies in primary prevention. Screening should be reserved for those high-risk patients exposed to industrial hazards or those unable to stop smoking.

CHEST X-RAY

Previous studies have demonstrated that screening for lung cancer by annual chest x-ray does little to reduce cancer mortality. Eighty percent of patients with x-ray evidence of lung cancer had negative x-rays 1 year previously [6]. More frequent x-rays may increase the detection rate but will not decrease mortality. In a 10-year study of 6,136 men over age 45 screened by semiannual chest x-ray, one-half of all cancers were detected by x-rays. The 5-year survival rate, however, was similar to the nonscreened population [2].

SPUTUM CYTOLOGY

Examination of exfoliated cells appearing in the sputum has been useful as a means of detecting early disease. A close correlation exists between positive sputum cytology and the presence of lung cancer. When four to five specimens are obtained, there is up to 100-percent sensitivity [2]. Fifty thousand cytologies were studied from a group of 6,000 uranium workers. Those patients with abnormal sputum samples gradually developed invasive carcinoma. Abnormal sputum cytologies require further diagnostic studies, which until recently have not been able to localize the lesion. Better diagnostic procedures, such as fiberoptic bronchoscopy with the use of toluidine blue bronchial

spray to highlight abnormal areas of mucosa, broncho-
grams, and biopsies, have improved the localization of
early lesions. In a series of 360 cases of lung cancer, 84
percent were visualized by bronchogram and bronchoscopy [3]. Despite the utility of sputum cytologies, cytology is tedious, expensive, and requires a skilled cytologist
for interpretation.

CHEST X-RAY AND CYTOLOGY

Combining the two accepted screening procedures of chest
x-ray and cytology has improved early detection of lung
cancer. An early report from the Mayo Clinic's Lung Project, part of the National Cancer Institute's Early Lung
Cancer Cooperative Group, has shown that it is possible to
detect lung cancer at a curable stage by alternating cytology and chest x-ray every 4 months. Although the Mayo
experience is limited, the screening program has demonstrated an ability to detect early, presymptomatic lung
cancer. More than 70 percent of newly detected cases were
resected "for cure." Long-term follow-up is necessary to
determine whether survival, not just earlier detection, has
been improved. Patient acceptance has been high, with 90
percent of patients remaining in the program [7].

Theoretically, aggressive application of lung cancer
screening by chest x-ray and cytology could increase the
5-year survival rate among lung cancer patients to nearly
50 percent [3]. Based on these findings, preliminary
though they may be, it seems that the principal hope for
the high-risk individual is participation in a screening program combining sputum cytology and chest x-ray with the
hope that either cancer cells will be found in the sputum
or a tumor will be found on the chest x-ray when surgical
treatment is still possible [3].

ARYL HYDROCARBON HYDROXYLASE

Early work with aryl hydrocarbon hydroxylase suggests
that this enzyme may be associated with increased suscep-

tibility to bronchogenic carcinoma. The use of aryl hydro-carbon hydroxylase as a screening procedure is not yet clinically applicable [6].

Prevention

Since smoking is the major etiological factor in lung cancer, prevention must be directed at reducing smoking behavior and reducing the risk of those who continue to smoke.

SMOKING MODIFICATION

Smoking cessation is a complicated phenomenon. A number of different programs, techniques, and products are available to aid a smoker to quit. Since there is no active way to compare outcome results between programs, selecting among a variety of programs and products may produce real difficulties. Often the "help-stop-smoking industry" takes advantage of the situation to manipulate their outcome data to attract more customers. It is quite likely that the specific technique adopted is not nearly as important as the motivation of the individual smoker to quit. No technique is universally acceptable, and all have some disadvantages. Findings from previous studies, however, have revealed several generalized principles that may help the physician evaluate the different programs. The more successful programs have incorporated the following points [9]:

1. Positive orientation—Stopping smoking is not an act of deprivation, but rather an act of gaining control of one's life.
2. Assuming responsibility—The individual must assume responsibility for his own smoking behavior. Treatment can aid the patient to quit but can never cause him to quit. Education, advice, and supportive action cannot by themselves make a patient quit smoking. The program must emphasize individual responsibility.

3. Contact continuity—The development of a personal relationship with the therapist is important in encouraging a patient to quit smoking.

4. Unimportance of the specific quitting technique—The type of treatment received may be minor compared to the individual motivation. Almost all techniques "work" if followed. One technique, however, may work better for some than for others.

5. Action—Quitting within about 14 days should be encouraged in the program.

6. Importance of maintenance—The first 3 months after treatment are critical for the recent ex-smoker. This is the period during which 90 percent of recidivism occurs. Thus, an effective program must continue support through this period.

7. Weight control—One of the major concerns of individuals contemplating quitting is that they will gain weight by substituting food for cigarettes. Treatment programs must acknowledge this common fear and deemphasize its importance. Few people, when quitting smoking, actually gain significant weight that remains for any period of time. Nutritional information can be provided about smoking substitutes low in calories. Individuals who persist in weight worries should be referred to a nutritional program if significant weight gain occurs. As a result of these measures, one study of 2,520 people showed that only 5 percent actually experienced weight gains over 5 pounds [11].

Another difficulty of smoking cessation programs has been that most existing programs offer one standard approach. No regard is given to individual differences in either personality or degree of addiction. Some smokers can stop merely with the guidance and urgings of a friend, family member, or physician. On the other hand, some smokers probably can never stop. A specific level of intervention should be matched to specific smoking characteristics. The American Health Foundation is currently attempting to identify the amount and type of aid needed by individual smokers [11].

Level 1 or minimal intervention programs are applied to those not motivated to stop smoking. Assuming that most adults already acknowledge that smoking is harmful to health, the goal of level 1 intervention is to make the particular smoker aware that smoking has a personal meaning for him and that there is value to be gained from stopping. A physician can deliver this message in the usual doctor-patient setting. Preliminary analysis of 2,000 persons showed an overall success rate of approximately 8 percent.

Level 2, or intermediate intervention, involves utilization of audiovisual aids at the patient's own convenience in helping the smoker to stop. A variety of aids and books are currently available. Two such titles are *Learning to Live Without Cigarettes* by William A. Allen, Gerhard Angermann, and William Faekler (Doubleday, Garden City, N.Y., 1973) and *You Can Quit Smoking in 14 Days* by Walter Ross (Reader's Digest Press, New York, 1974). Initial results with this level of intervention reveal that one-half of the participants dropped out and never completed the required study course. The overall success rate for this level was 19 percent after 1 month.

Level 3 or maximal intervention programs provide not only a structured procedure for quitting, but also the support of a therapist or of a group who are also trying to quit. Included in this level are structured programs, group counseling, individual counseling, and hypnotic intervention. After 1 year, all these methods produced approximately a 25-percent success rate in abstention and a 40-percent rate of smoking reduction.

Level 4 or intensive programming intervention is currently an experimental level that uses techniques that either are more demanding of participants or use drugs or nicotine substitutes.

The primary care physician can start a patient at level 1 and progress as necessary to level 3. Most primary care physicians will probably assume responsibility for level 1 and 2 programs. Level 3 programs are often conducted by others. For those physicians interested in utilizing some of the techniques of smoking cessation, however, the following discussion will present some of the specific techniques that are currently utilized in level 3 programs.

Any particular smoking cessation program may utilize one or more of the following methods:

1. Substitute activity—For many smokers, activities such as chewing gum, sucking cinnamon, playing with matchsticks and so forth satisfy the need to keep their hands busy and receive oral stimulation. Many readily available, socially acceptable substitutes for the missed activity will do.
2. Dosage reduction—This method utilizes a gradual reduction in the amount of each cigarette smoked, the degree of inhalation, and the number of cigarettes smoked.
   a. Reduced cigarette length—After recording a baseline number of cigarettes smoked per day, the smoker marks each cigarette with a felt pen at the midpoint. Smoking beyond the midpoint is not permitted. Clearly it is important that the rate of puffing, frequency of smoking, and degree of inhalation do not change. The half-smoked cigarettes may be collected as evidence of compliance, if necessary.
   b. Decreased degree of inhalation—Deep inhalers should be asked to practice inhaling less deeply.
   c. Decreased frequency of smoking per day—Generally smokers are able to reduce gradually the number of cigarettes smoked per day. This technique works best over an extended period of time.
3. Situational and event control—Many persons smoke on a reflex basis, i.e., first thing in the morning, while having a cup of coffee, or while watching television. This type of habitual smoker can break the automatic response by making the cigarette less accessible or by having only a certain place to smoke. Any activity that causes him to think about the cigarette before lighting it may allow him to minimize use.
4. Relaxation, deep breathing—Since smoking may serve to reduce tension, a substitute relaxation technique may aid cessation efforts. A variety of relaxation methods are available that increase awareness of muscles, both in relaxation and in stress. Eventually, a relaxed muscle state can be produced at will.
5. Buddy system—Ex-smokers can be an important asset to others attempting to quit. A buddy can provide individual support during difficult times. The responsibility of being a buddy may further increase motivation to maintain abstinence.
6. Rapid smoking technique—The rapid smoking technique is an aversive conditioning technique that produces a noxious "overdose" through continuous and rapid smoking. Each aversive

conditioning session consists of one puff every 6 seconds and continues until the subject is either unable or unwilling to smoke at the required pace. This produces symptoms similar to "nicotine poisoning," with increased heart rate, increased blood pressure, and hyperventilation. Since cardiac arrhythmias may be induced, however, the procedure is a risk to other than healthy persons. Nevertheless, this technique claims a success rate of up to 60 percent at 6 months.

Other programs may utilize individual treatment, individual therapy, group therapy, or hypnosis. Although techniques using hypnosis have claimed the highest success rates, with up to 88-percent abstention at 1 year, the population tested was very small and the results may therefore be misleading. In addition, this method requires a one-to-one therapist-patient ratio, making it less cost-effective. Currently used antismoking drugs have no demonstrated pharmacological effect in making it either more difficult to smoke or less difficult to stop. Their use, therefore, at this time is experimental.

LESS HAZARDOUS CIGARETTE

The less hazardous cigarette provides an immediate benefit to all smokers. The cigarette that delivers the least tar and nicotine and has the lowest specific carcinogenic activity is the least hazardous. These qualities are influenced by the type of tobacco, plant culture, curing, blending, tobacco additives, and filtration. Popular cigarettes on the market today range from a low of 8 mg of tar to a high of 19 mg. Over the past 10 years, the average tar and nicotine content of cigarettes has decreased by 30 percent [8]. Further reduction is essential.

Summary and Recommendations

The primary care physician must adopt an aggressive two-prong approach to lung cancer prevention. He can (1) attempt to motivate all his patients to eliminate or at least reduce the hazards of smoking, and he can (2) establish screening programs for high-risk groups, e.g., men over age 45 who are persistent smokers or who are exposed to known industrial carcinogens.

RECOMMENDATIONS

1. Smoking modification—Lung cancer mortality could be virtually eliminated by eliminating smoking. Smoking modification programs have variable, but often impressive results. Although no studies have demonstrated the potential effectiveness of the primary care physician in motivating patients to attend and complete a smoking modification program, it is likely that the physician could play an influential role. At the least, all smoking patients should be encouraged to participate in a suitable program.
2. Reducing the risk—Despite repeated warnings about its effects and the almost universal awareness of the health hazards, smoking continues relatively unabated. Persistent smokers can reduce their risk by smoking less and by smoking cigarettes lower in tar. Efforts to identify smokers who are highly susceptible to lung cancer are promising, but conclusive means are not yet available.
3. Lung cancer screening—Although primary prevention is a preferable means of reducing lung cancer mortality, screening programs for high-risk groups are effective. Persistent smokers and workers exposed to asbestos, uranium, nickel, chromate, and arsenic should be offered a screening program involving sputum cytology and chest x-ray. Although there is some preliminary evidence that people living in areas close to certain industries are at higher risk, their risk has not been sufficiently documented to warrant screening. Urban dwellers are also at higher risk, but neither is it practical nor is the risk great enough to warrant general screening.
4. Public health approach—Although the public health approach has had little success, the primary care physician could support school health-education programs, antismoking campaigns, and legislative efforts to lower the tar content of cigarettes. Finally, he can provide an example to his patients by personally not smoking.

References

1. Beamis, J., A. Stein, and J. Andrews. Changing epidemiology of lung cancer. *Med. Clin. North Am.* 59 :315, 1975.

2. Benfield, J. Current and future concepts of lung cancer. *Ann. Intern. Med.* 83 :93, 1975.

3. Berlin, N. Early detection and localization of bronchogenic carcinoma. *Chest* 67:508, 1975.

4. Blot, W., and J. Fraumeni. Arsenical air pollution and lung cancer. *Lancet* 2:142, 1975.

5. Blot, W., and J. Fraumeni. Geographic patterns of lung cancer: Industrial correlations. *Am. J. Epidemiol.* 103:539, 1976.

6. Brooks, S. Early detection of lung cancer in high risk populations. *J.O.M.* 17:19, 1975.

7. Fontana, R. et al. The Mayo lung project for early detection and localization of bronchogenic carcinoma: A status report. *Chest* 67:511, 1975.

8. Gori, G. Smoking and cancer: Research in the etiology and prevention at the National Cancer Institute. *Cancer* 30:1340, 1972.

9. Hunt, W., and D. Besplec. An evaluation of current methods of modifying smoking behavior. *J. Clin. Psychol.* 30:431, 1974.

10. Newhouse, M. Asbestos in the work place and the community. *Ann. Occup. Hyg.* 16:97, 1973.

11. Shawchuk, L. Smoking cessation programs of the American Health Foundation, *Prev. Med.* 54:57, 1976.

12. Wynder, E. Etiology of lung cancer. *Cancer* 30:1332, 1972.

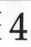

Colorectal Cancer

Occurrence

Colorectal cancers represent 15 percent of all cancers and, except for cancer of the lung, are the most common cause of cancer deaths in the United States, accounting for fifty thousand deaths annually. In 1975, the one hundred thousand new reported cases represented the second largest increase in cancer incidence for any cancer site. Colorectal carcinoma is the fifth leading cause of death in the 60- to 64-year age group (Fig. 4-1). It has been estimated that up to two-thirds of the deaths from colorectal carcinomas could have been prevented by routine screening procedures.

Risk Factors

DIET
All present evidence indicates that cancers of the colon and rectum, like other cancers, are related to environmental factors [10]. Tumors of this site are more common in the United States and Western countries than in Japan and underdeveloped countries. British workers in Africa noted the striking rarity among rural black of colonic cancer, polyps, diverticulosis, and appendicitis. Other

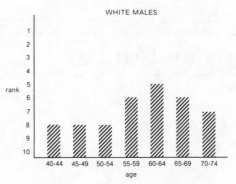

Figure 4-1. *Rank of colorectal carcinoma as cause of death by age.*

ethnic groups in Africa who ate Western-style diets had these disorders in frequencies approaching those of Westerners.

Epidemiological analysis has postulated that the crucial difference between the life-styles of the rural blacks and the more westernized groups was diet, in particular the amount of fiber and roughage in the diet [1]. Further epidemiological evidence from the United States shows that colorectal cancers are less common among lower socioeconomic groups (particularly blacks) whose major caloric intake is from carbohydrates. Carbohydrates provide more fiber than the diets higher in fats and protein eaten by higher socioeconomic groups.

Dietary fiber refers to all ingested foods that reach the large intestine essentially unchanged. A wide variety of plants, whose stored carbohydrates and cell walls, such as cellulose, lignin, and some polysaccharides, are resistant to the digestive enzymes of the small intestine, provide fiber content. Table 4-1 lists the dietary fiber in selected foods.

Since all dietary fiber reaches the colon, the colon is most affected by fiber. Fiber will affect colonic motor function, bacterial flora, and metabolic products. The result of increasing dietary fiber to 50 gm per day will

Table 4-1. Dietary Fiber in Selected Foods

Food	Total Dietary Fiber (gm/100 gm)
All Bran	26.7
Puffed Wheat	15.41
Wholemeal bread	8.50
Peas, frozen (raw)	7.75
Peanut butter	7.55
Beans, baked (canned)	7.27
Carrot, young (boiled)	3.70
Potato (raw)	3.51
White bread	2.72
Peaches (whole)	2.28

Source: Adapted from D. Southgate, *J. Hum. Nutr.* 30:303, 1976.

increase the weight of the stool from 80 to 150 gm per day to 250 gm per day. Continued passage of stools of this increased volume implies a dilution effect of potential carcinogens, as well as increased absorptive capacity for postulated carcinogens. In addition, since the larger fecal content is expelled more rapidly, there is less contact time between the postulated carcinogens and the colon [5].

The basic hypothesis of increased fiber content is evolutionary. For millions of years man has principally consumed a diet of vegetables, which are high in dietary fiber. Only recently has there been a change to more refined carbohydrates, fat, and animal proteins.

Some workers postulate the rate of the stool as being "protective." Although dietary fiber is not currently regarded as an essential nutrient, some minimal intake, perhaps over 30 gm per day for an adult, may be beneficial and "protective." Children should be taught to eat a diet high in fiber and low in sugar, salt, and fat.

POLYPS

A polyp is any mass of tissue protruding into the lumen of the bowel. Approximately 5 to 10 percent of the adult population has one or more polypoid lesions. Polyps can be divided into three major classes: (1) *neoplastic,* including adenomatous and villous polyps, which are associated with an increased risk of developing colorectal carcinoma; (2) *hamartomas,* including juvenile polyps and polyps in the Peutz-Jeghers syndrome, which do not become neoplastic, and hemangiomas, which may possibly become neoplastic; and (3) *inflammatory,* as seen in ulcerative colitis [9].

Hereditary Polyposis. Familial adenomatous polyposis carries a high risk of developing into colorectal carcinoma. It is transmitted by a dominant gene and appears in 40 percent of the offspring of an affected family. Without prophylactic treatment, cancer will develop in almost 100 percent of patients with familial adenomatous polyposis. Familial polyposis is usually detected in childhood as a result of colonic symptoms.

Adenomatous Polyps. In the absence of a hereditary polypoid disease, the malignant potential of an isolated adenomatous polyp is uncertain but is related to its size. In adenomatous polyps less than 1.5 cm in size, the risk of developing invasive carcinoma is approximately 2 percent. Since operative morbidity and mortality approaches 2 percent, polyps of this size warrant close periodic observation rather than surgery. Newer techniques of removal through the colonoscope, which have lower complication rates, may well be justified. Polyps greater than 2.0 cm are routinely removed. Polyps that double in size in less than 6 months are also routinely removed, since the risk of carcinoma increases to 30 percent in these rapidly growing polyps.

Villous Adenomas. Villous adenomas are sessile polyps that most frequently appear in the rectum and sigmoid colon and have a high malignant potential. In a series of 261 patients with villous adenomas followed over a 30-year period, 51 percent remained benign. Forty-two percent became carcinomas in situ, and 33 percent became frankly invasive carcinomas [9].

Ulcerative Colitis. Patients with ulcerative colitis have an increased risk of developing colorectal cancer. The risk of neoplastic degeneration increases with the duration of the disease. After 10 years of ulcerative colitis, approximately 10 to 20 percent of patients will develop colorectal carcinoma. The risk is greater for those who were under 20 years old when the ulcerative colitis started or in whom the entire colon is involved. Colorectal carcinoma rarely develops in localized proctosigmoiditis.

Diagnosis and Screening

At the time of diagnosis, most patients with cancer of the colon are beyond cure and will die of their disease despite the most intensive and aggressive treatment. The overall 5-year survival rate for all cases of colorectal carcinoma is currently 40 percent. More extensive surgery, more aggressive chemotherapy, or more widespread radiotherapy will not increase the rate of cure. Earlier diagnosis can increase the cure rate by detecting lesions when they are in an early, quiescent phase more amenable to treatment. Mass screening programs for lesions of the gastrointestinal tract have proved to be a valid approach. In Japan, mass screening surveys for gastric cancer in asymptomatic patients resulted in increased detection rates of very early lesions and in cure rates as high as 90 percent.

Six major diagnostic procedures are available for detecting colorectal cancers: (1) examining the stool for occult blood, (2) sigmoidoscopy, (3) clinical examination, (4) barium enema, (5) colonoscopy, and (6) immunological markers. Because a screening test has to be reasonably sensitive and able to pick up early presymptomatic lesions in addition to being safe, simple, and acceptable, only the first two procedures, examining the stool for occult blood and sigmoidoscopy, may be suitable for mass screening programs.

OCCULT BLOOD

Most patients with colorectal carcinoma will have blood in their stool. Thus, examination of the stool for occult blood is widely recommended as an aid to early diagnosis. Several currently available techniques exist.

A comparative evaluation of guaiac solution, orthotoluidine tablets, and guaiac-impregnated filter paper (Hemoccult) showed that the Hemoccult was the least sensitive of the three tests. A minimum of 25 ml of blood or 5 mg of hemoglobin per 1 gm of stool was required to produce a positive test. Nevertheless, the Hemoccult was highly reproducible and virtually eliminated false positive results. In addition, 28 percent of initially negative guaiac solution and orthotoluidine tests became positive after storage. Only 2 percent of initially negative Hemoccult tests became positive after storage. Because of the reliability and stability of Hemoccult, it is currently widely recommended as an effective screening technique.

False negatives, although they may occur, can be decreased. Random testing of a single stool specimen is inadequate and will lead to many false negative findings. To decrease the false negative rate, Greegor developed a screening protocol designed to stimulate bleeding from existing lesions. A meat-free, high-roughage diet is eaten for 4 days. After the first day, 2 aliquots of each of three separate stools are tested for occult blood by guaiac-impregnated filter paper. A subsequent analysis of the six-stool guaiac protocol suggested that further testing beyond two Hemoccults yielded little in the way of increased sensitivity (i.e., decreased false negatives) [6].

The test is not specific for colorectal carcinoma. Other bleeding lesions will be detected. In a series of 900 asymptomatic patients, 5 percent were positive for occult blood; 1 in 5 of these had a carcinoma.

Although lesions can be detected early by this method, asymptomatic patients may find it difficult to follow a meat-free, high-bulk diet for 4 days. Dietary instructions can be optional. The physician can decide whether prior instructions regarding a meat-free, high-bulk diet with avoidance of peroxidase-producing vegetables, such as horseradish and turnips, should be given.

All patients over the age of 40 should be given three slides, an envelope addressed to the doctor's office, and an instruction sheet of how to prepare the slides (Fig. 4-2). Most patients will not object to the preparation of the slides. Office personnel rarely show reluctance to handle these slides compared to traditional stool specimens.

SIGMOIDOSCOPY

The use of sigmoidoscopy as a screening procedure is controversial. Its proponents claim that two-thirds of deaths from colorectal carcinomas could be prevented by routine sigmoidoscopy exams [7]. Other proponents suggest that virtual elimination of lower bowel cancer is possible with the use of the sigmoidoscope [4]. A look at the data is impressive.

In a series from the Memorial Sloan-Kettering Cancer Center, 47,000 sigmoidoscopy exams on 26,000 asymptomatic patients were performed. One case of colonic cancer was detected for every 450 exams [8]. Of the colonic cancers detected, there was an 88-percent 5-year survival rate, which is far better than the 40-percent average 5-year survival rate. Although the pickup rate of malignant lesions is relatively low, polyps were found in 5 to 10 percent of all patients. The finding and removal of polyps may also be important in decreasing the risk of developing colorectal carcinoma. In a 25-year study of

ROUTINE

Hemoccult slides are routinely used to check the intestinal tract for microscopic amounts of bleeding. Follow the directions below, and return the test slides to this office.

1. Write your name, address, and the date the specimen was collected in the space provided on each slide.
2. Collect a small stool specimen on one end of the applicator.
3. Apply a thin smear inside the patient side of the slide.
4. Prepare one slide from three consecutive bowel movements.
5. Do not collect specimens during menstrual periods or while suffering from bleeding hemorrhoids.
6. Protect the slides from heat, fluorescent light, and sunlight.

SPECIAL DIAGNOSTIC DIET

Start the diet at least 48 hours before collecting the first stool specimen. Remain on the diet until all the stool specimens have been collected. During the test period

1. Eat no rare meat, turnips, or horseradish.
2. Do not take any medicine, tonic, or vitamin preparation that contains aspirin or vitamin C (ascorbic acid) in excess of 250 mg per day.
3. Eat plenty of vegetables, both raw and cooked.
4. Eat plenty of fruit, especially prunes, grapes, plums, and apples.
5. Eat moderate amounts of peanuts and popcorn each day.
6. Include a bran-containing cereal in your daily diet.

If any of the above are known from past experience to cause gastrointestinal symptoms, please notify this office.

Figure 4-2. Sample patient instructions for using Hemoccult slides.

18,000 patients who had normal sigmoidoscopy exams, 85 percent of the statistically expected adenocarcinomas did not develop. Polyp removal is considered the significant factor of the low cancer incidence. Each of the cancers that did appear was found early and was well localized to the bowel wall.

Opponents of sigmoidoscopy as a routine screening procedure claim it is costly and time-consuming, is occasionally hazardous, requires a special skill, and is unpleasant for the patient. Various estimates have been made of the cost of uncovering a malignant lesion. In a study of 1,900 sigmoidoscopies in a family practice, the average cost of uncovering a malignant-prone individual or a malignant disease was $800 [7]. Some estimate that 10,000 examinations would have to be done to produce seven additional 5-year survivals. At the Cancer Detection Center at the University of Minnesota, each sigmoidoscopy took 6 minutes of the physician's time. A more conservative estimate for the average physician seems to be 15 minutes. In a series of 103,000 sigmoidoscopy examinations, five perforations occurred. There is no known report of a death secondary to a perforation. Nor is there any known report of a sudden death during the sigmoidoscopy exam either from an acute myocardial infarction or from a pulmonary embolus. Although a certain degree of skill is required in performing a sigmoidoscopy, this can readily be taught to all physicians. Even if only 20 cm can be visualized through the sigmoidoscope, 65 percent of all tumors can be seen. If only 15 cm can be visualized, 50 percent of all tumors can be seen.

The consensus is that annual sigmoidoscopy, by itself, is not the answer to mass screening for colorectal carcinoma. A more selective use of sigmoidoscopy according to known risk factors seems to be a rational compromise. Patients can be selected by prior, more simple tests, such as for occult blood in the stool, or by the presence of diseases associated with an increased risk of colorectal carcinoma.

Since more than 90 percent of colorectal cancer deaths occur in persons over 52 years of age, age 50 or even 45 is an appropriate time for the initiation of periodic exams. Colorectal cancer has a slow growth rate, the doubling time being approximately 3 years. Thus a sigmoidoscopy examination every 2 to 3 years can adequately detect most curable carcinomas. A longer interval may also be satisfactory, since no patient who has discontinued annual examinations has developed colorectal cancer within the first 7 years following examination.

For optimal sigmoidoscopy results, the rectosigmoid should be properly prepared 4 to 5 hours before the examination. Cleansing enemas should be given until returns are clear. Only physiological solutions should be used. Hypotonic or hypertonic solutions or irritants such as soap may cause erythema that will interfere with proper interpretation of the findings. If the examination is performed too soon after the enemas, excess mucus may still be present that may also interfere with interpreting the findings.

The proper technique for sigmoidoscopy begins with a digital examination of the rectum. The digital exam will insure the absence of any obstruction that would make insertion of the rigid sigmoidoscope dangerous. At this time, the complete digital examination of the anal canal and lower rectal ampulla, and prostate gland for men, can be carried out (see Chap. 7 under the heading Physical Examination for technique).

The knee-chest position is most satisfactory for sigmoidoscopy. Several examination tables are available that conveniently allow the patient to be examined in this position. If no such table is available and if the patient is strong enough, the knee-chest position on a regular table or bed is adequate. If the patient cannot tolerate this position, Sims's position (left lateral position) is the best alternative.

The patient should be adequately draped to minimize exposure of the buttocks and genitalia. An explanation of the procedure as it proceeds will also help alleviate anxiety.

Next, lubricate the sigmoidoscope with the obturator in place, and insert it gently into the anus, aiming toward the umbilicus. Once past the anal canal (5 cm), remove the obturator. Attach the lens and light. Under direct visualization, gradually insert the scope past Houston's valves. Occasional inflation with the rubber bulb may be necessary to open and pass through the valves. At a depth of approximately 16 cm, a sharp turn to the patient's right marks the beginning of the sigmoid colon. Changing the angle of the sigmoidoscope will aid in engaging the tip of the tube into the sigmoid colon. The scope should never be forced. It is better to be satisfied with lesser distance than to risk a perforation. When the scope is inserted as far as it will go, it is gradually withdrawn. Inspection of the entire lumen as the scope is withdrawn is then performed.

CLINICAL EXAMINATION

Clinical examination is an inadequate screening technique because it fails to detect early lesions and cannot detect the majority of bowel cancers. Signs and symptoms appear relatively late in the course of the disease. Once patients become symptomatic, one-half are beyond cure. Even the dogma that the majority of rectal cancer is within the reach of the examining finger has been challenged. Only 12 percent of all bowel cancers and only 30 percent of all rectal cancers extend to within 6 cm of the anal margin [1].

BARIUM ENEMA

The barium enema is the standard method of diagnosing cancer above the peritoneal reflection. Except for cancer of the rectum, it is 90 percent accurate. Its cost, time, and radiation exposure preclude its use as a routine screening technique.

COLONOSCOPY

Fiberoptic colonoscopy is used to detect lesions beyond the reach of the sigmoidoscope. Clinical studies have shown that this technique is useful in examining selected patients at high-risk for colorectal carcinoma. Because colonoscopy is time-consuming and relatively difficult to perform even by experienced physicians, it is not suitable for mass screening of asymptomatic patients. Colonoscopy is, however, assuming a major role in the aggressive management of high-risk patients. Polyps can be snared through the scope without abdominal surgery. Biopsies and cytologies of suspicious lesions can be done. As the distribution of colonic lesions changes, with more and more lesions being located beyond the reach of the sigmoidoscope, use of the colonoscope will increase. Complete reliance on sigmoidoscopy as the major endoscopic technique will lessen. Indications for colonoscopy are [2]

1. X-ray negative, with continued colonic symptoms.
2. X-ray questionable, for further diagnostic studies.
3. X-ray positive, with one radiologically proven lesion before a limited surgical resection; other lesions should be searched for either pre- or intraoperatively.
4. High-risk groups.
5. Follow-ups.

IMMUNOLOGICAL MARKERS

Carcinoembryonic antigen (CEA), a fetal protein, was discovered in 1965 and originally thought to be specific for colonic adenocarcinoma. Subsequently, the antigen has been found in association with a history of heavy smoking, with other cancers, particularly lung and ovarian, and with a host of other diseases, such as ulcerative and granulomatous colitis, diverticulitis, cirrhosis, pancreatitis, and benign breast diseases [8]. An isomeric species of carcinoembryonic antigen, CEA-S, has been reported to be a more specific marker for colonic carcinoma [3]. Its persistent lack of specificity and its high rate of false positives, however, preclude its use as a screening tool. Carcinoembryonic antigen is currently useful in measuring the clinical progression of and response to treatment. Other biochemical markers will need to be discovered to make this a useful screening technique.

Summary and Recommendations

Although the etiology of colorectal carcinoma is un-known, epidemiological and clinical studies have identified risk factors and high-risk patients. High-meat, high-fat, and low-bulk diets are associated with higher rates of colo-rectal cancer. Certain polyp-forming diseases as well as ulcerative colitis are also associated with a higher risk of developing colorectal carcinoma. Intensive, periodic in-vestigation of patients with these risk factors will certainly prove beneficial.

An additional high-risk group should be selected by mass screening of asymptomatic patients at risk (e.g., those over 40 years of age). Testing stools for occult blood and routine sigmoidoscopies are appropriate. Those tests with positive results should be followed with an aggressive diagnostic approach, including sigmoidoscopy (if not al-ready done), colonoscopy, blood CEA, and some of the newer techniques now being developed such as fluorescent exfoliative rectocolonic cytology.

RECOMMENDATIONS

1. Diet—Although the evidence is not conclusive, the bulk of
   evidence suggests a strong association between colorectal carcinoma and high-meat, high-fat and low-bulk diets. A prudent
   reduction of meat and fat in the diet with an increase in bulk
   would be beneficial in decreasing the risk not only of colorectal
   carcinoma but also of arteriosclerotic cardiovascular disease.

2. Occult blood—Because of the relative ease and great potential benefit of identifying a high-risk population for colorectal cancer, all adults over age 40 should have yearly stool examinations for occult blood. One sample from each of three different stools is recommended for testing.
3. Sigmoidoscopies—Sigmoidoscopies every 3 years in adults over age 45 have greatly decreased mortality from colorectal carcinoma. It is not clear whether yearly screening for occult blood obviates the necessity for periodic sigmoidoscopy exams. Because of the small but significant false negative rate associated with occult blood examinations, it might still be prudent to supplement them with periodic sigmoidoscopies, especially if the Greegor protocol was not strictly adhered to. Further studies in this area are required.
4. High-risk patients—All high-risk patients, whether at high risk because of polyps, associated diseases, or positive screening tests, require intensive follow-up.

References

1. Berg, J., and M. Howell. The geographic pathology of bowel cancers. *Cancer* 34:807, 1974.
2. Davis, C. Fiberoptic colonoscopy—Early diagnosis of colorectal cancer. *J. Med. Assoc. Ga.* 64(1):18, 1975.
3. Edginton, T., R. Astarita, and E. Plow: Association of an isomeric species of carcinoembryonic antigen with neoplasia of the gastro-intestinal tract. *N. Engl. J. Med.* 293:103, 1975.
4. Gilbertsen, V. Proctosigmoidoscopy and polypectomy in reducing the incidence of rectal carcinoma. *Cancer* 34:936, 1974.
5. Mendeloff, A. Dietary fiber and human health. *N. Engl. J. Med.* 297:811, 1977.
6. Neuhauser, D.; and A. Lewick. What do we gain from the sixth stool guaiac? *J. Engl. J. Med.* 293:226, 1975.
7. Rasgon, I. Value of proctosigmoidoscopy in colo-rectal carcinoma. *J. Fam. Pract.* 2(2):95, 1975.
8. Sherlock, P., and S. Winawer. Modern approaches to early identification of large bowel cancer. *J. Dig. Dis.* 19(10):959, 1974.
9. Stauffer, J. Polypoid Tumors of the Colon. In M. Sleisenger, *Gastrointestinal Diseases.* Saunders, Philadelphia, 1978.
10. Wynder, E., and B. Reddy. The epidemiology of cancer of the large bowel. *J. Dig. Dis.* 19(10):937, 1974.

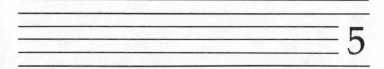

Breast Cancer

Occurrence

Despite improvement in the overall mortality figures for women in the United States, breast cancer continues to be one of the leading causes of mortality for women over 30 years of age (Figs. 5-1, 5-2). The average American woman has a 7- to 8-percent chance of developing breast cancer sometime in her life. Breast cancer is by far the most frequent site of female cancer, being two times as frequent as cancer of the cervix, the next leading cancer site. The death rate from cancer of the breast has increased from 14.6 deaths per 100,000 in 1968 to 15.2 deaths per 100,000 in 1975 (Fig. 5-3).

Etiology

Because the etiology of breast cancer remains obscure, no clinically useful preventive program can be advocated. An understanding of the etiological factors currently considered important, however, serves to identify potentially useful preventive measures. Emphasis has been placed upon the role of oncogenic viruses in the etiology of breast cancer [5, 7]. Although the origin, transmission,

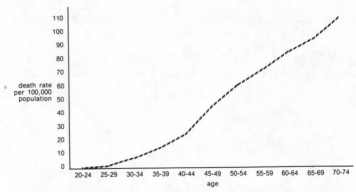

Figure 5-1. *Death rate by age from breast cancer, 1975.*

and significance of viral infection in humans has not been
established with the same certainty as it has been in animals, the evidence is strongly suggestive of the importance
of the virus in human disease. In spite of incomplete
knowledge about the importance of viral infection in
humans and the exact route of transmission, one author
advises complete abstinence of breast-feeding of infants
in families with a history of breast cancer on the assumption that the virus may be transmitted through breast
milk.

Many of the presumed significant factors in breast cancer
etiology may have a genetic component. The hormonal

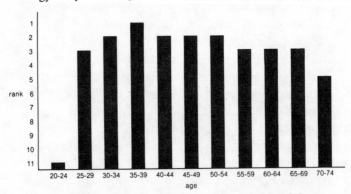

Figure 5-2. *Rank of breast cancer as cause of death by age.*

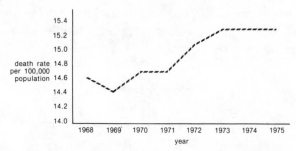

Figure 5-3. Death rate by year from breast cancer.

milieu in which breast cancer develops may be genetically determined. The high risk of women who have relatives with breast cancer suggests a genetic influence. Perhaps as important, genetics may be responsible for determining resistance to the virus or for regulating host defenses.

Hormones, particularly estrogens, once considered the main carcinogenic factors, are now considered to be strong carcinogenic promoters. Irradiation may cause cancer by direct toxic effects on the cell. Other less well documented and understood carcinogenic influences have also been studied but at this time have little clinical significance. Dietary fats appear to affect the development of breast cancer by possibly affecting the production of carcinogenic estrogens from intestinal bacteria. Chronic psychogenic stress may exert carcinogenic potential by depressing immune responses.

Although the concensus is that breast cancer is a multifactorial disease, the central observation for clinical preventive medicine is that the initial events of malignant change take place early in life. A widely discussed 1959 study from Guernsey Island noted that decreased urinary androgen excretion is present for many years in patients who initially were clinically normal but who subsequently developed breast cancer. More recent work has emphasized the protective effect of estriol, which is present in high amounts during pregnancy and may explain the protective effect of pregnancy. In order for estriol to be protective, it must be present at a young age, presumably when noxious agents are most active.

Risk Factors

Although the search for a cause of breast cancer has not led to a means of prevention, several hypotheses have linked breast cancer to specific characteristics of women. The following characteristics may define a high-risk population [5]:

1. Multiple primary cancers.
   a. Previous breast cancer—Women with cancer in one breast may subsequently develop a second primary carcinoma in the opposite breast. Bilateral primary breast cancer is relatively common. Rates of bilaterality range from 4 percent up to 20 percent. A recent review suggested that 7 to 10 percent of women with breast cancer eventually developed cancer in the opposite breast.
   b. Endometrial or ovarian cancer—Cancer of both the breast and the endometrium occurs in the same women with a greater than chance frequency. Women with cancer of the endometrium have a breast cancer risk 1.3 to 2.0 times that of the general population. The risk of developing a second tumor is greatest within the first few years of the appearance of the first. Although less well established, ovarian cancer and cancer of the breast have also been associated.
2. Family history of breast cancer—Relatives of women with breast cancer have two to three times the general population's breast cancer rate. The risk is as great for paternal as for maternal relatives. It has been suggested that relatives of women with bilateral breast cancer have three times the risk of developing breast cancer than do relatives of women with unilateral disease.
3. Other breast disease—Women with chronic cystic mastitis have about four times the breast cancer rate of normal women. This extra risk persists as long as 40 years after the initial diagnosis. Acute breast conditions associated with lactation are not associated with increased risk of breast cancer.

4. No children before age 35—There exists an inverse relationship between the risk of breast cancer and parity.
   a. Women parous before age 18 have one-third the breast cancer risk of women whose first delivery is delayed until after age 35.
   b. Pregnancy must occur before age 30 to be protective.
   c. The protective effect is limited to full-term pregnancies and to the first birth.
   d. Protection may last until age 75 or older.
5. More than 35 years of menstrual history.
   a. Early menarche—Women with menarche before age 16 have 1.8 times the risk of those with later menarche.
   b. Late menopause—Women with late natural menopause (age 55 or older) have twice the risk of women whose menopause occurred before age 45.

The definition of a high-risk population identifies those who would most benefit from screening. Survival is clearly related to stage at the time of initial diagnosis. Earlier detection in larger numbers of women will decrease overall mortality. In a series of patients from Presbyterian Hospital, women with 5-cm lesions had approximately a 70-percent incidence of axillary metastases, compared to women with 1-cm lesions, who had a 40-percent incidence of axillary metastases [3]. The 5-year clinical cure rate in patients without axillary metastases in this series was over 90 percent.

Screening

Four major approaches to earlier detection of breast cancer are currently available: periodic breast self-examination, periodic clinical examination, thermography, and mammography. An optimal screening program for the general population and for high-risk patients remains controversial. Since the primary care physician is in an ideal position to coordinate and integrate the approach to prevention, he must be familiar with the advantages and limitations of each screening method.

BREAST SELF-EXAMINATION

Reports that up to 90 percent of all breast malignancies were discovered by patients themselves have fostered the recommendation that breast self-examination should be the primary approach to early detection. Data from the Preventive Medicine Institute–Strang Clinic, however, suggest that self-examination should be considered as only one among several screening tests, each having its own limitations, sensitivity, specificity, and optimal frequency of application [11]. While this may be so, it is likely that teaching women how to examine their own breasts correctly may yield the greatest possible gain in early diagnosis. A correct technique for self-examination greatly increases a woman's chance of detecting a lesion in her own breast. Many discoveries of breast lesions are accidental, often made during the course of casual palpation while bathing. If women were taught to examine their breasts regularly, systematically, and with correct techniques, improvement in early diagnosis would naturally result.

Breast self-examination is most effective in detecting cancers in women under age 45. A recent study that evaluated the roles of self-examination, clinical examination, and mammography in early tumor detection in young women revealed that patients detected 84 percent of tumors themselves. Physical examiniation by physicians detected 14 percent of tumors. Two percent were detected by mammography [4]. In young women, breast cancers are frequently palpable before they can be visualized by present radiographic techniques. Thus, self-examination and clinical examination are the most successful methods for early detection in this age group.

Primary care physicians must clearly capitalize on their potential to instruct and motivate their patients to perform regular breast self-examinations. Only a small fraction of women regularly and routinely perform breast self-examinations. Estimates of women who do perform periodic self-examination range from 5 percent of a general population to 37 percent of those attending a breast disease clinic, a more select and more motivated group. A recent study showed that person-to-person health education could increase regular breast self-examination practices to 70 percent of a population [2]. General fear of cancer, mass media publicity, and the individual guidance of a physician influence breast self-examination practices.

Breast self-examination is best performed once a month after completion of the menstrual period, when breast engorgement is at a minimum. In addition, some physicians recommend examining the breasts during routine bathing, as the hand glides easily over wet skin. Since this may tend to produce an abnormal fear of cancer in some women, the physician must individualize his recommendations.

Breast self-examination includes inspection and palpation (Fig. 5-4). To detect a change in the shape of the breasts, a woman must inspect both breasts in front of a mirror with her arms at her side. Next, the woman raises her arms high over her head and looks for changes in contour, swelling, dimpling of the skin, or changes in the nipples. A similar inspection is made while resting the palms on the hips and then pressing firmly to flex the pectoral muscles. The left breast normally may be slightly larger than the right. Regular inspection, however, will determine normal variations in a particular woman.

Palpation is best done in the supine position, with the shoulder on the side being examined slightly elevated. This helps flatten the breast against the chest wall. The fingers of the opposite hand are used to palpate. The inner half of the breast is palpated with the arm raised and the outer half with the arm at the side.

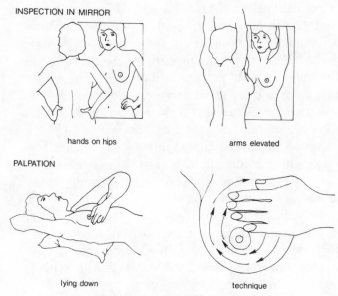

INSPECTION IN MIRROR

hands on hips   arms elevated

PALPATION

lying down   technique

Figure 5-4. Breast self-examination.

Soft palpation is done with the tips of the fingers moving in concentric circles. When the breast is examined by the patient herself in this manner, it is not uncommon for tumors as small as 1 cm to be recognized.

CLINICAL EXAMINATION

With the exception of skin tumors, tumors of the breast are the most accessible to early diagnosis. The family practitioner, the internist, and the obstetrician/gynecologist in particular have the opportunity to examine patients' breasts during the course of routine, periodic examinations. In addition, they have the opportunity to examine the breasts during the course of treatment for unrelated problems. It is the responsibility of the physician, maintaining a constantly high index of suspicion based upon incidence and mortality data, to periodically examine the breasts. Adequate examination of the breasts requires a separate step in the physical examination. Undoubtedly, lesions are missed by a cursory passing of the hand over the breast on the way to examining the heart or lungs. A proper examination is "a well ordered procedure including different steps and requiring ten to fifteen minutes even when no abnormality is found" [3].

It is desirable to follow a set routine for examining the breasts to avoid overlooking important details.

1. Inspection of the breasts—With the patient stripped to the waist and sitting facing the examiner, the examiner carefully inspects the breasts, first with the patient's arms at her side, then with the arms raised, and then with the arms pressed against the hips. A comparison of the contour of both breasts, their relative height on the chest wall, and their relative size is made. Bulging, dimpling, peau d'orange, nipple retraction, or unilateral, dilated superficial veins may denote underlying disease.

2. Supraclavicular and axillary regions—In order to examine the axilla, the pectoral muscles must be relaxed. This is achieved by the examiner's supporting the patient's arm on his arm and then palpating with the tips of the fingers of his other hand. The number, consistency, and movability of nodes are noted. Lymph nodes high in the axilla or nodes lying close behind the pectoral muscle are difficult to feel and are easily missed. Unfortunately, palpation is inaccurate for determining whether nodes contain metastases. In one series in which the examiner thought nodes were not involved, 44 percent were found to contain metastases at surgery.

3. Palpation—Palpation is best performed with the patient supine and with a small pillow placed under the shoulder of the breast being examined. This helps flatten the breast against the thorax. In palpating the medial half of the breast, it is advisable to have the patient's arm raised above her head to provide a flatter surface. In palpating the lateral half of the breast, it is advisable to have the patient's arm at her side. Since breast tissue may often extend over a wide area, palpation must range from the midline of the sternum medially to the lower edge of the clavicle superiorly to the edge of the latissimus dorsi laterally, including the axillary tail. Gentle palpation with the flat of the fingers in a systematic fashion is the most informative approach. Although many prefer to palpate in concentric circles, I prefer walking the flats of my first two fingers up and down as if "mowing a lawn."

Clinical examination can detect early breast tumors not detected by other screening procedures. In a study of 20,211 women aged 40 to 64, 132 breast cancers were detected on screening. Fifty-nine were diagnosed as a result of clinical examination alone, 44 by radiographic evidence alone, and 29 by both clinical and radiographic methods [9]. If the clinical examination had been omitted, 45 percent of the breast cancers would not have been detected. In the 40- to 49-year age group, 61 percent of the cases would have been missed. Routine clinical breast exams of all female patients over 25 years of age are an important means of breast cancer detection. In a series of breast cancer cases, almost 5 percent were initially detected by routine examination of patients who came to the physician for totally unrelated complaints.

Although clinical examination is safe, reasonably effective, and acceptable to most patients as a screening technique, it has the disadvantages of being expensive in terms of the physician's time and subject to a high rate of false negatives. For physicians to detect a breast lesion as early as palpation permits, ideally they should examine their patients every 3 months. Physicians cannot provide this service for most women [12].

It should be recognized that evaluation of the breast presents one of the most difficult problems facing the primary care physician. The principal problems in clinical examination are in detecting small lesions in difficult-to-examine breasts and in differentiating the small nodule that requires biopsy from mastitis. Even if a high index of suspicion is maintained, errors will be made. Clinical examination failed to detect lesions in 33 percent of patients with radiographically diagnosed breast tumors. When the examining physicians had the opportunity to reexamine these patients with the knowledge of the radiographic findings, the detection rate increased by 50 percent.

Montgomery, Bowers, and Taylor developed a set of rules to aid the clinician evaluate the breast. While they were developed before the advent of mammography, they have withstood the test of time and serve as practical guidelines. Their verbatim recommendations are as follows [6] :

1. *There is some safety in numbers: to wit, bilateral diffuse induration of the breast is rarely cancerous and offers no site of selection for biopsy. Such cases should be observed periodically.*
2. *Cancer may appear in an area of chronic mastitis by coincidence, or possibly as a result of cause and effect. Any local change of texture or development of a "dominant" lesion should therefore be biopsied promptly.*
3. *Unilateral persistent fibrocystic disease, such as appears frequently in the upper and outer quadrant of the breast, should be freely excised and studied in multiple section.*
4. *Enlarged glands of the axilla adjacent to such areas of induration should also be excised for study, even though the breast area itself is benign.*
5. *In the case of patients appearing with a well defined mass in the breast, arrangements should be made for prompt biopsy and mastectomy at the same sitting if the tissue is positive.*
6. *In a slender undernourished woman, the whole fabric of the breast may be revealed to a degree suggesting fibrocystic disease or even small neoplasms.*
7. *Lipoma-like masses in the breast of aged women often harbor scirrhous carcinoma. Be strongly suspicious of any lesion of the breast after the menopause, especially if there is no hormone therapy.*
8. *Questionable areas of nodulation in the breasts of pregnant women should be biopsied under local anesthesia, the biopsy examined in paraffin section, and the definitive therapy carefully planned.*
9. *Small apparent lesions of the breast discovered at examination just before menstruation should be rechecked after the period is over; they may disappear.*
10. *Minute and doubtful lesions which seem scarcely deserving of biopsy even though they persist after the period should be rechecked every 6 to 8 weeks until the problem is resolved.*
11. *The patient with serous discharge from the nipple should be biopsied whenever the secretion can be traced or when-*

ever induration is palpable at any point around the areola or adjacent breast tissue.

12. *A patient with fibrocystic disease may have to be biopsied several times in the course of years to satisfy the physician that cancer is not developing. In some such cases, simple mastectomy becomes the ultimate solution.*

13. *The patient who complains most of pain is least likely to have carcinoma, unless she has an enormous lesion.*

14. *The patient with extensive fibrocystic disease or adenosis of the breast, and a strong family history of cancer, had better have a simple mastectomy.*

15. *Postmenopausal patients should be discouraged in the prolonged use of estrogens because of the untoward effect on the breasts.*

THERMOGRAPHY

Thermography, the technique of pictorally representing infrared radiation, is based upon a comparison of heat patterns between breasts. A breast cancer is hotter than its surroundings, and the temperature of the venous blood supply leaving a cancer is greater than its arterial supply. Thermography was initially thought to meet many of the requirements of an ideal screening procedure. Although the cost of equipment is high, the technique is inexpensive to perform. It is simple and quick, can be repeated at frequent intervals, and is acceptable to a majority of women. It is safe and without radiation hazard. Abnormal thermograms indicate the need for further investigation.

In spite of the advantages of thermography, the procedure lacks specificity. The false positive rates are often increased by benign conditions or even anatomical variations simulating the thermographic signs of cancer. Less of a problem, but also troublesome, is the false negative rate. Not all cancers are "hot." Scirrhous carcinomas, for example, are almost always cold. A thermogram of a woman with bilateral cancer may be interpreted as negative because of the lack of a temperature differential between the breasts. Furthermore, difficulty in interpreting thermograms occurs with women who have recently started taking oral contraceptives, with women who have large, pendulous breasts that do not cool properly, and with some women just before menses when there is a more prominent venous pattern.

Few studies to date have objectively determined the value of thermography as a screening procedure. In one study of 4,621 asymptomatic women over 35 years of age, 628 (13.6%) had abnormal thermograms [10]. These were further investigated by mammography, with the following results:

Patients	Results of Mammography
42	Positive for malignancy with biopsy recommended
62	Suspicious for malignancy, to be followed
326	Abnormal but negative for malignancy
198	Negative

The relatively high rate of false positives (high sensitivity, low specificity) limits the use of thermography to initial screening. The lack of specificity precludes its use in differential diagnosis, but when combined with historical and clinical information, it has been successful in determining which patients should be considered for mammography.

More recently it has been suggested that the use of thermography as a single modality of screening is not warranted. Among experienced thermographers, the false positive rate was so high, while the true positive rate was so relatively low, that thermography was of little use in identifying patients with early cancers that could not be detected by other methods. The role of thermography in a screening program in conjunction with physical examination and mammography is controversial and requires further objective study.

MAMMOGRAPHY

The first clear-cut estimate of the benefits of mammography came from the HIP Study in which 62,000 women between the ages of 40 and 64 years were paired and randomly divided between a control group (no extra attention) and a study group offering a breast screening program (medical history, clinical examination, and mammography). There was one-third lower mortality in the study group, with one-third of the cancer cases being detected by mammography alone. The benefits of mammography in increasing survival are more difficult to estimate, but from 20,000 women and 65,000 sets of mammograms, from 12 to 14 cancer deaths were avoided.

The potential cost in radiation damage must be weighed against these benefits. Abundant experimental and clinical data have linked ionizing radiation with breast cancer. The average dose of radiation delivered to the breast during mammography depends upon the machine, the image receptor, and the method used. The average dose in the HIP Study was 7.7 rads. Another study showed the average dose of a six-film series ranged from 4.88 to 7.5 rads. The dose was considerably lower with the use of a four-film series and with the use of newer techniques. The use of xeromammography permits a dosage reduction of up to 50 percent. The absolute risk of radiation exposure has been estimated as six cases of breast cancer/million women /rad.

Although the optimal use of mammography in screening well women is not known, certain inherent features of mammography offer the primary care physician a rational approach to its use. Mammography is most accurate in women over 50 years of age. In the older women, adipose tissue replaces breast parenchyma, and masses become more easily detected radiographically. Thermography is less productive in women under 35 years of age because premenopausal breast parenchyma produces a dense radiographic pattern that obscures underlying disease and because breast cancer has a lower incidence in this age group.

Although the optimal interval between exams for well women is not known, many experts agree that a baseline examination should be performed on patients between 35 and 40 years of age. *Indications for initial radiographic examination of the breast,* regardless of age, are [8]

1. High-risk patients
2. Contemplated breast surgery
3. Palpable mass
4. Large, difficult-to-examine breasts
5. Cancerophobia
6. Other breast complaints, e.g., dimpling, skin thickening, retraction
7. Metastases with an unidentified primary site

Indications for serial radiographic studies are

1. Prior breast cancer—Examination of the opposite breast is recommended 6 months after surgery and every year thereafter.
2. Strong family history of breast cancer.
3. Breast dysplasia.
4. Previous equivocal mammograms.

Summary and Recommendations

Because of the persistently high rate of deaths from breast cancer, the primary care physician must coordinate a rational approach to early breast cancer detection among women. Observations have demonstrated that malignant changes take place early in life. Progress is being made in identifying suitable markers for those malignant changes that will eventually lead to breast cancer. In the meantime, the most sensitive and specific procedure for detecting early breast cancer is the three-way screen: clinical examination, combined with thermography and mammography. It is generally agreed that the three-way screen should be limited to high-risk women.

Less definitive information is available on the screening

Preventive Primary Medicine

of normal-risk women. The following recommendations, by taking into account the known advantages and limitations of each screening procedure, are an attempt to present a feasible guideline to early breast cancer detection for normal-risk women.

RECOMMENDATIONS FOR SCREENING WELL WOMEN

1. Identification of high-risk patients.
   a. Medical history can help in identifying high-risk patients. Sixty-two percent of an unselected population of supposedly well women over age 35 turned out to be at greater risk for breast cancer.
   b. In addition to high-risk patients, patients with difficult-to-examine breasts should be identified for close follow-up.
   c. Nursing mothers with a strong family history of breast cancer should be cautioned about possible transmission of breast cancer to their infants through a virus that may be present in breast milk.
2. Palpation.
   a. All women should be taught and motivated to perform breast self-examinations.
   b. All women over age 25 should have at least annual clinical breast examinations.
3. Thermography.
   a. The place of thermography in routine screening of well women is controversial.
   b. Most experts limit thermography, when combined with clinical examination and mammography, to high-risk patients.
4. Mammography.
   a. A baseline mammogram at age 35 to 40 is recommended by many experts.
   b. Optimal interval screening of well women is uncertain. Serial mammograms for normal-risk women are not optimally beneficial until after age 50.

References

1. Bailar, J.   Mammography: A contrary view. *Ann. Intern. Med.* 84:77, 1976.
2. Gastrin, G.   New techniques for increasing efficiency of self-

examination in early diagnosis of breast cancer. *Br. Med. J.*
11 (6038):745, 1976.

3. Haagensen, C. *Carcinoma of the Breast: A Monograph for Physicians.* American Cancer Society, New York, 1968.

4. Lesnick, G. Breast cancer in the young woman. *J.A.M.A.* 237:967, 1977.

5. MacMahon, B. and P. Cole. Etiology of human breast cancer: A review. *J. Natl. Cancer Inst.* 50:21, 1973.

6. Montgomery, T., P. Bowers, and H. Taylor. Breast lesions. *Obstet. Gynecol.* 1:394, 1953.

7. Papaioannou, A. N. Etiologic factors in cancer of the breast in humans. *Surg. Gynecol. Obstet.* 138:257, 1974.

8. Sadowsky, N. Radiologic detection of breast cancer: Review and recommendations. *N. Engl. J. Med.* 294:370, 1976.

9. Stark, A., and S. Way. The use of thermovision in the detection of early breast cancer. *Cancer* 33:1664, 1974.

10. Stark, A., and S. Way. The screening of well women for the early detection of breast cancer using clinical examination with thermography and mammography. *Cancer* 33:1671, 1974.

11. Thiesson, E. Breast self examination in proper perspective. *Cancer* 28:1537, 1971.

12. Venet, L. et al. Adequacies and inadequacies of breast examinations by physicians in mass screening. *Cancer* 38:1546, 1971.

Cervical Cancer

Occurrence

Although there has been a decrease in mortality from cervical cancer in the United States over the past 20 years, cervical cancer continues to be a major public health problem, accounting for thirteen thousand deaths annually (Fig. 6-1). Cervical cancer is the second most common site of female cancer, exceeded only by cancer of the breast. Two percent of women reaching age 80 will develop cervical cancer. Cervical cancer is a controllable disease. It has been stated that if every woman at risk had a Papanicolaou (Pap) smear regularly, cancer of the cervix could be prevented [10].

Etiology

The overwhelming bulk of evidence supports the hypothesis that cervical cancer is a venereal disease in which a carcinogen is transmitted during coitus. Herpesvirus type 2 has been postulated to be the initiating or promoting carcinogenic agent that can be transmitted during coitus by a male donor to a female host at risk [6, 7]. Based upon epi-

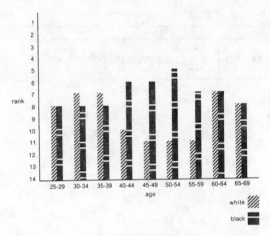

Figure 6-1. Rank of cervical cancer as cause of death by age and race.

demiological and biological evidence, an association exists between genital herpes and cervical cancer. Biologically, the virus has oncogenic potential. It causes tumors in frogs, fowl, and monkeys and has been associated with naso-pharyngeal carcinoma and Burkitt's lymphoma in humans. The virus is transmitted venereally. Infection may result in either an acute, self-limited condition or in a latent persistence of the virus that may predispose to subsequent malignant transformation. Epidemiologically, a tumor-specific, complement-fixing antibody was detected in 90 percent of cases of invasive cervical carcinoma, in 68 percent of cases of carcinoma in situ, and in only 5 percent of controls. Epidemiological studies also demonstrate a greater incidence of cervical abnormalities among women with proven herpetic infection of the genitalia than among control women. The association, although strong, is not causal. It is still unknown whether herpesvirus infection precedes cervical neoplastic changes or whether herpesvirus infection and cervical cancer are covariables of sexual activity.

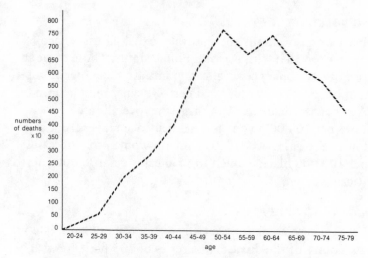

Figure 6-2. Deaths by age from carcinoma of the cervix.

Risk Factors

Although the exact cause of cervical cancer is unclear, several risk factors have been identified [8, 9].

AGE
Cervical carcinoma has a peak incidence in women in their 40s and 50s. It rarely occurs in women under 20 years of age (Fig. 6-2).

EARLY ONSET OF COITUS
Women who begin coitus during adolescence, before age 17, have 1.4 times the risk of developing cervical cancer than do women who begin later.

MULTIPLE SEXUAL PARTNERS
Sexual intercourse with increasing numbers of partners increases the risk of cervical carcinoma. Women who have more than one male sexual partner increase their risk by 80 percent.

SOCIOECONOMIC STATUS

Early onset of coitus and multiple sexual partners have been associated with socioeconomic status. Those most at risk of developing cervical carcinoma are the indigent population, particularly blacks, Puerto Ricans, and Mexican Americans. Incidence data suggest an overall rate of 14.9 cases per 100,000 women. The incidence ranges from a low of 3.6 cases per 100,000 Jewish women to 47.8 cases per 100,000 black women to 97.6 cases per 100,000 Puerto Rican women.

SIGNS AND SYMPTOMS

Cervical carcinoma is essentially asymptomatic until late in the course of the disease. In a series of 135 patients with carcinoma in situ, 46 percent had no symptoms. However, several conditions, mostly coincidental, are associated with cervical carcinoma. Thirty percent of patients had abnormal bleeding of some kind, and 24 percent had leukorrhea.

OTHER FACTORS

Although several other factors have previously been implicated in the etiology of cervical carcinoma, a recent review of the epidemiological studies failed to find any association between cervical carcinoma and coital frequency, abortions, pregnancy and deliveries, menstrual patterns, contraception, or noncircumcision of sexual contacts [8].

Screening

Most of the evidence suggests that a continuum exists between cervical dysplasia, carcinoma in situ, and invasive carcinoma. The more severe the dysplasia, the more likely it is to progress [6]. Most, but not all, intraepithelial lesions progress to invasion. Some may regress. In a study to determine the factors related to cytological progression of cervical atypia, 539 women with cytologically diagnosed

cervical dysplasia underwent long-term follow-up [5].
After 5 years, the overall probability of progression from
dysplasia to carcinoma in situ was 41.2 percent. The highest rate of progression occurred in the first 6 months after
the initially atypical smear. If the follow-up smear was also
atypical, there was a 25-percent chance of progression. If
there was a negative follow-up smear, the chance of progression dropped to 2 percent. The progression rates were
highest in the 30- to 44-year age group.

Cervical cancer detection programs are based upon the
principle of a continuous progression of cervical dysplasia
to carcinoma in situ to invasive carcinoma. Such an association has been demonstrated clinically, morpholog-
ically, and epidemiologically [2]. Cytological screening of
women will detect the disease in its earliest stages, so that
the risk of subsequent invasive carcinoma is eliminated.
Although the role of cervical cytology in reducing the incidence of invasive carcinoma is strongly suggested, the
incidence rates have been decreasing since 1947, even before the advent of mass screening programs. It is possible
that since many of the risk factors are associated with
lower socioeconomic status, an increase in the overall standard of living may have contributed to a decrease in the
incidence rates of cervical carcinoma.

In an attempt to study the effect of screening in decreasing morbidity and mortality from cervical carcinoma,
a population with an organized screening program was
compared to a control population with no organized program [1]. The fall in death rates in the screened population far exceeded that in the control population. The
greatest decreases were in the 30- to 39-year age group,
with a decrease of 70.8 percent, and in the 50- to 59-year
age group, with a decrease of 69 percent.

The Pap smear is at best a sample of cells exfoliated or
scraped onto an applicator. The collection technique directly affects the diagnostic yield. Obtaining a proper specimen is essential to correct diagnosis. So many different

methods have been devised for obtaining cells for cytological study that the procedure may seem relatively confusing. However, only a few basic guidelines need to be followed. A satisfactory specimen must contain an adequate number of well-preserved epithelial cells. Sampling from the squamocolumnar junction increases sensitivity, particularly from the younger age groups. Obtaining two smears increases the detection rate of abnormal cytology by 86 percent [9]. In one study, initial cytology detected only 50 percent of patients with abnormalities. In a study of 2,823 Pap smears taken in a family planning service, it was found that obtaining two smears considerably increased the detection rate [13].

Besides a scanty or unrepresentative sample of cells, other factors may influence cytological interpretation. Poorly processed or dried specimens cause cellular distortion and misinterpretation. Infections, particularly trichomonas vaginitis, cause nuclear atypia. Squamous metaplasia, the replacement of exposed columnar epithelium by squamous epithelium, may produce less differentiated cells.

A number of conditions may hinder diagnostic interpretation. A specimen can be obtained at any time, as long as it is properly taken. Sampling during active menstrual flow yields a higher percentage of unsatisfactory specimens. However, menses may be the only time cancer cells are shed. Although douching within 24 hours of the examination may alter the vaginal pool, very little change is made in the endocervical specimen. Rather than frequently postpone the Pap smear for minor reasons, it is usually best to obtain a smear when the opportunity arises and repeat it if indicated.

A Pap smear can have several uses, which may influence the particular technique used for obtaining the specimen. Only specimens obtained for detecting carcinoma of the cervix are described here.

The cervix is exposed with an unlubricated bivalve speculum. Abundant clear mucus is removed from the cervix

with a ring forceps prior to smear taking. Mucus is obtained from the posterior vaginal pool with the spatula
(Fig. 6-3A). It is then placed upon the slide as a thick drop
(Fig. 6-3B). The pointed end of the wooden spatula is inserted high up into the endocervical canal and rotated a
full turn (Fig. 6-3C). Pressure is maintained against the
edge of the spatula to obtain a sample from the squamocolumnar junction. The cellular material is then transferred
to the slide and mixed with the lower portion of the vaginal pool mucus drop (Fig. 6-3D). The drop is then smeared
with a light stroke of the spatula (Fig. 6-3E). Immediate
wet fixation yields the highest diagnostic accuracy. The
simplest procedure is to drop the wet slide into 95% ethyl
alcohol. Some commercial spray fixatives are also satisfactory if applied immediately.

In the patient over 40 years of age, the squamocolumnar
junction has often receded within the endocervix and may
be out of reach of the wooden spatula. A saline-moistened,
nonabsorbent, cotton-tipped applicator can be used in
these cases to obtain the endocervical smear. Cytology is
not meant to be diagnostic. It can only point to the cervix
as the site of abnormality. In a study to compare cytology
with a formal tissue diagnosis, the cytologist's opinion was
compared to a final tissue diagnosis in a series of 338 patients from Columbia University [10]. When the cyto-
pathologist reported dysplasia, only 56 percent of patients
actually had dysplasia. A few had invasive carcinoma, some
had carcinoma in situ, and some had no pathology. Negative cytological findings were particularly common in mild
or moderate dysplasia. With a cytological diagnosis of carcinoma in situ, 68 percent of patients had the same tissue
diagnosis. Most of the remainder had dysplasia; some had
invasive carcinoma. With a cytological diagnosis of invasive
carcinoma, only 19 percent actually had invasive carcinoma.
Most had carcinoma in situ or dysplasia. In addition, there
were 9 percent false negatives.

The yield of screening programs depends upon the target

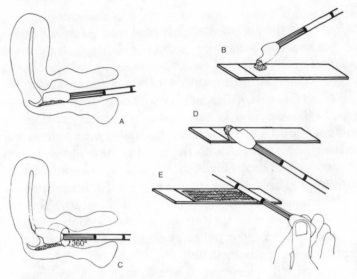

Figure 6-3. Papanicolaou smear technique.

population. In indigent populations, approximately one out of every hundred smears will be atypical. In higher socioeconomic populations, approximately one out of every thousand smears will be atypical. In a series of 53,350 Pap smears from a university clinic with a mixed population, 7.3 lesions were detected from every 1,000 Pap exams [10]. The success of screening programs has been greatest in the younger age groups, with a falloff after age 45. A recent poll conducted by the American Cancer Society in an urban area showed that 78 percent of the female population over age 21 had had a Pap test at least once. Almost 100 percent of the women under 30 had been screened [1]. A survey of 16,435 Pap smears conducted by the Massachusetts Department of Public Health also showed that the younger age groups were better screened. Only 44 percent of smears were performed on women over age 35 [4].

Since 97.5 percent of all deaths from cervical carcinoma occur in the over-35 age group and since the death rate increases steadily with age, are the wrong women being screened? Not necessarily so. Because the greatest useful-ness of cervical cytology has been in the determination of cancer in its earliest stages of development, screening of the younger population represents a useful approach. Screening younger women makes possible the identifica-tion of patients at risk with cervical dysplasia (25–35 years of age) and the identification of patients with carcinoma in situ (35–45 years of age). The early treatment of patients with dysplasia and carcinoma in situ is responsible for de-creasing the subsequent death rate from invasive cervical carcinoma. Nevertheless, screening the older women is also important in detecting carcinoma in its earliest stages and in decreasing the death rate from invasive and metastatic cervical carcinoma.

The frequency of repeating Pap smears depends upon the rate cervical dysplasia progresses to carcinoma in situ to invasive carcinoma and upon the false negative rate. Most experts agree that it may take up to 15 years for dysplasia to progress to invasive carcinoma. The false negative rate, the number of times the Pap smear misses actual pathol-ogy, is approximately one out of ten. Because of this sig-nificant false negative rate, it is safer to repeat the Pap smear frequently. It is probably ideal, especially in the high-risk patient, to repeat the Pap smear every 6 months. However, the frequency of routine cytopathological ex-aminations must be individualized. Because of the slow progression rate of cervical carcinoma, longer intervals are acceptable. The interval for any asymptomatic patient following negative examination and with a negative history may fall between 6 months and 2 years. The actual interval chosen may depend upon such risk factors as age, parity, previous disease, and socioeconomic status.

THE ABNORMAL PAP SMEAR

The reporting system for the Pap smear is based upon the following five classes:

Class	*Cytological Description*
1	Normal
2	Atypia—inflammatory atrophy, metaplasia
3	Mild, moderate, severe dysplasia
4	Carcinoma in situ
5	Invasive carcinoma

Most cytologists simplify this classification into three major subdivisions: normal, class 1 or 2; abnormal, class 3 or 4; and positive for malignancy, class 5.

Until recently, smears that were persistently class 3 or worse were indications for conization. The expense, inconvenience, and the 7- to 15-percent complication rate of conizations can now be drastically reduced by the proper use of endocervical curettage and colposcopically directed biopsies.

Colposcopy is an examination of the cervix magnified up to 50 times through the viewing microscope. Colposcopic examination, best done by an experienced colposcopist, is performed during a 3- to 5-minute period, with applications of acetic acid to enhance the colposcopic pattern. If the full extent of the lesion cannot be visualized under the colposcope, endocervical curettage is performed. Directed biopsies are taken of all suspicious areas noted on colposcopy.

Endocervical curettage and colposcopy have reduced the need for diagnostic conizations by 85 percent [3]. Endocervical curettage is more reliable in diagnosing neoplasia than endocervical smears. The colposcope can determine the exact area of the cervix causing the atypical smears. A prospective study of 76 patients with negative endocervical scrapings found that the colposcope was over 90-percent accurate in detecting the abnormal area on the cervix [14]. Another series of 603 patients with atypical Pap smears supports the belief that a negative endocervical scraping allows exact diagnosis by the colposcope. It is now believed that Pap smears, colposcopically directed biopsies, and endocervical curettings, when used as a unit, can establish an accurate outpatient diagnosis comparable to conizations [11].

Summary and Recommendations

Despite a 20-year decrease in cervical carcinoma mortality, cervical cancer still ranks as the second most common cite of female cancer. Although the etiology is unknown, biological and epidemiological evidence demonstrates an association between herpesvirus type 2 and cervical cancer. Epidemiological studies have also identified early onset of coitus, multiple sexual partners, and low socioeconomic status as high-risk factors. The decline in mortality is generally credited to widespread Pap screening programs. It is believed that application of the screening program to all women at risk will further decrease mortality.

RECOMMENDATIONS

1. The primary physician should periodically screen all women over age 20 as soon as they become sexually active.
2. A Pap smear every 6 months is probably ideal, especially for the sexually active or high-risk patient. A yearly screen is a reasonable alternative. Consecutively negative smears lessen the need for annual smears.
3. To increase sensitivity, two Pap smears may be obtained.
4. In class 2, benign atypical smears, treatment of the cervicitis may be indicated, and the Pap smear should be repeated in 6 months.
5. Class 3 smears should be repeated. If the repeat smear is class 1 or 2, it should be repeated again in 3 months. If that smear is again class 1 or 2, it should be repeated at 6-month intervals.
6. Persistent class 3 or worse smears require further diagnosis. The use of endocervical scrapings and colposcopically directed biopsies will decrease the need for diagnostic conizations.

References

1. Christopherson, W. et al. Cervical cancer control: A study of morbidity and mortality trends over a 21 year period. *Cancer* 38:1357, 1976.
2. Cramer, D. The role of cervical cytology in the declining morbidity and mortality of cervical cancer. *Cancer* 34:2018, 1974.
3. DePetrillo, A. et al. Colposcopic evaluation of the abnormal Papanicolaou test in pregnancy. *Am. J. Obstet. Gynecol.* 121:441, 1975.
4. Duffy, B. Papanicolaou testing: Are we screening the wrong women? *N. Engl. J. Med.* 294:223, 1976.
5. Hulka, B. and C. Redmond. Factors related to progression of cervical atypia. *Am. J. Epidemiol.* 93:23, 1971.
6. Kessler, I. Perspectives on the epidemiology of cervical cancer with special reference to the herpes virus hypothesis. *Cancer Res.* 34:1091, 1974.
7. Melnick, J., E. Adam, and W. Rawls. The causative role of herpes virus type 2 in cervical cancer. *Cancer* 34:1375, 1974.
8. Rotkin, I.D. A comparative review of key epidemiological studies in cervical cancer related to current searches for transmissible agents. *Cancer Res.* 33:1353, 1973.
9. Rubin, P. Cancer of the cervix. *J.A.M.A.* 193:212, 1965.
10. Shingleton, H. Evaluation of patients with atypical Pap smears. *Ala. J. Med. Sci.* 9:248, 1972.
11. Shingleton, H., H. Gore, and J. Austin. Out patient evaluation of patients with atypical Papanicolaou smears: Contribution of endo-cervical curettage. *Am. J. Obstet. Gynecol.* 126:122, 1976.
12. Schulman, J., and A. Hantz. The Pap smear: Take two. *Am. J. Obstet. Gynecol.* 121:1025, 1975.
13. Schulman, J., M. Lezton, and R. Hamilton. The Papanicolaou smear: An insensitive case finding procedure. *Am. J. Obstet. Gynecol.* 120:446, 1974.
14. Townsend, D., et al. Abnormal Papanicolaou smears: Evaluation by colposcopy and endo-cervical curettage. *Am. J. Obstet. Gynecol.* 108:429, 1970.

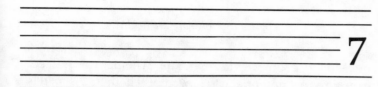

Prostatic Cancer

Occurrence

Carcinoma of the prostate is a common disease in aging men. In the United States, the overall incidence of 16.5 cases per 100,000 rises to 500 cases per 100,000 for men in the 75- to 79-year age group [9]. Mortality from prostatic carcinoma, second only to carcinoma of the lung, has been steadily increasing from 17.3 deaths per 100,000 in 1968 to 18.6 deaths per 100,000 in 1975. Men have a 2-percent lifetime risk of developing clinically significant carcinoma of the prostate [7].

Risk Factors

Despite the considerable risk of developing carcinoma of the prostate, there are few ways to define a high-risk group. The epidemiological studies on this disease are often conflicting and have given few clues to its etiology [3, 5, 7, 12, 14].

AGE

Prostatic carcinoma is rare in men before age 50, but its rate of incidence increases rapidly until age 80 and then increases at a somewhat slower rate. Whether this reflects exposure to a potential carcinogen or whether this merely reflects a direct or indirect consequence of aging is unclear.

RACE

Most epidemiological attention has focused on the wide differences in incidence rates among different races. In the United States, prostatic carcinoma is more common in blacks than in whites. Internationally, the yellow races, particularly the Japanese, have the lowest rates. An increased incidence among Japanese who migrate to this country suggests that the differences may be related to an unknown environmental factor [12].

HEREDITY

One study suggests a higher frequency of prostatic carcinoma in relatives of patients with the disease than in relatives of controls [5].

SEXUAL FACTORS

There is no general agreement on an association between sexual factors and carcinoma of the prostate. Two studies found the highest rates in widowed and divorced men [5, 7]. Married men, especially married men with children, had higher rates than did single men [5]. Sexual factors may account for these differences. Because another study found no differences in incidence between married and single men, the association between sexual factors and prostatic carcinoma is doubtful [12].

HORMONES

There is no direct relationship between steroid hormones and the development of prostatic carcinoma [3]. Although hormones act to stimulate prostatic epithelium where malignant changes may occur, they play no role in actual carcinogenesis. As is well known in treatment, hormones can affect the growth and development of prostatic cancer. Patients with cirrhosis have lower rates of prostatic cancer than patients with normal liver function. The inadequate removal of estrogens in cirrhotic patients presumably inhibits the growth of prostatic cancer.

OTHER FACTORS

A retrospective study of 300 patients with cancer of the prostate failed to show any association between prostatic carcinoma and socioeconomic status, alcohol or tobacco use, weight, height, blood group, or a history of benign prostatic hyperplasia [12].

Screening and Early Detection

When patients with prostatic carcinoma are first seen, many already have distant metastases or regional disease extending beyond the capsule. In a 10-year study of 500 patients with carcinoma of the prostate, the mean age was 69.3 years. At the time of initial diagnosis, 76 percent of these patients already had extensive carcinoma beyond the capsule. In only 24 percent of patients was the cancer confined to the prostate [9]. Autopsy evidence indicates that clinically inapparent lesions are at least twice as prevalent as clinically apparent lesions [11]. It has been estimated that as many as 35 percent of men over age 50 have innocuous microfoci of prostatic carcinoma [2].

The goal of early detection is to distinguish between those cancers that may remain indefinitely quiescent and require no therapy and those that may progress without early intervention. Recent studies on the natural history of prostatic carcinoma indicate that the cancer progresses from early stages, curable by local treatment, to stages of regional spread, with little chance of cure, to stages of dis-

tant metastasis, with no chance of cure, in approximately
4 years [13]. There is also evidence that, at least histo-
logically, the early stages of the disease are divided between patients with innocuous microfoci and patients
with potentially lethal tumors.

No screening test can satisfactorily detect potentially
lethal tumors at an early stage. Although physical examination has been the cornerstone of early detection, newer
biochemical and immunological techniques are necessary
to improve screening for prostatic cancer. Unsuspected
prostatic cancer remains a significant problem. In a series
of 887 patients who underwent suprapubic prostatectomy
for supposedly benign prostatic hyperplasia, 6.5 percent
had prostatic carcinoma detected by careful pathological
analysis of the specimens [1]. In another series of 891
supposedly normal patients, 5.8 percent had unsuspected
prostatic nodules [6].

PHYSICAL EXAMINATION
Rectal examination with subsequent biopsy of suspicious
areas is the only feasible method of early prostatic cancer
detection. A proper technique for rectal examination is
essential to increase diagnostic yield. Since it is difficult
to examine the size and landmarks of the prostate in a
patient with a full bladder, the bladder must be emptied
prior to a digital examination. The patient may be placed
in the dorsal lithotomy position, the left lateral prone
position, the knee-chest position, or the standing knee-
elbow position. In the last position, the examination may
be less painful if the feet are approximately 12 inches
apart, with the toes pointing inward. Having the patient
hold his breath will decrease anal sphincter tone and will
facilitate entry of a gloved lubricated finger.

The patient is then asked to strain as if to pass stool so
that the examiner can palpate hemorrhoids or polyps. The
presence of fissures or fistulas should also be noted. The

posterior wall is examined next for any abnormality.

Next, the anterior wall of the anus is examined. The prostate is a firm, smooth swelling in the anterior wall of the rectum. It resembles the shape and size of a chestnut and weighs approximately 20 gm. It is also described as heart-shaped, with the apex pointing toward the anal sphincter. It is divided by a shallow sulcus separating the lateral lobes. In enlarged prostates, the sulcus disappears. The lateral border of the prostate should be sharply demarcated from the surrounding tissues.

The prostate gland consists of five lobes, the median lobe, two lateral lobes, a posterior lobe, and an anterior lobe. The posterior lobe is the most common site for developing prostatic cancer. Frequently, prostatic cancer will start as a palpable hard nodule near the posterior surface of the gland. As it grows, the entire gland may become fixed, enlarged, and stony hard, or there may be several hard nodules.

The value of palpation in early prostatic cancer detection is limited, however, because many cancers develop without palpable findings. In a study of 1,134 patients where physical findings were compared to tissue diagnoses, 18.7 percent of patients with nonsuspicious prostates on physical examination turned out to have significant prostatic cancer as diagnosed by biopsy [6].

Even though many potentially curable prostatic cancers produce no nodularity or localized induration, the presence of a palpable nodule is significant. Nodules increase in frequency with age, from 0 percent in the fourth decade to 26 percent in the ninth decade. In a series of 1,134 patients, 52 percent of all nodules contained malignant cells [8].

Although one author recommends twice yearly prostate examinations for men over 50 years of age, no study has ever shown that frequent rectal examinations increase the detection of early localized disease [6].

BIOPSY

Since there is no absolute way to differentiate benign from malignant prostatic nodules by physical examination alone, all prostatic nodules must be suspect. The definitive diagnosis of carcinoma of the prostate must be made by biopsy, either open biopsy, needle punch biopsy, or aspiration biopsy.

Although the primary care physician may feel most comfortable referring all patients with prostatic nodules to a urologist for further evaluation, this may often be impractical. Needle aspiration biopsy may be suitable as a preliminary office screening procedure, particularly when multiple sites need to be biopsied. Aspiration biopsy will not interfere with the results of the usual needle biopsy. Therefore, following negative aspiration biopsy, needle punch biopsy can be done.

Aspiration biopsy is an office procedure that can be done following rectal examination. Anesthesia is not necessary because of the paucity of pain fibers in the rectum. A 20- or 22-gauge needle attached to a disposable 10-ml syringe is introduced rectally, advanced to the indurated area, and inserted into the prostate. The needle is rotated, then withdrawn under negative pressure, and a specimen is ejected onto an albuminized slide. A thin smear is made, fixed in 95% ethyl alcohol, and stained according to the method of the Papanicolaou smear.

Although aspiration biopsy has been widely used in other countries, it has not enjoyed widespread popularity here. Reports from Scandinavia stress its high reliability and safety. Up to 90 percent of prostatic carcinoma can be diagnosed by needle aspiration. There is good correlation between needle biopsy and aspiration biopsy. There are no false positive diagnoses. In contrast to the relatively high complication rate with punch biopsy, including hemorrhage, deep vein thrombosis, persistent tenderness and pain, and a need for catheterization following the procedure, there are no reported complications with needle aspiration biopsy. There have been no reports of tumor implantation following needle aspiration biopsy.

BIOCHEMICAL SCREENING

Measurement of the serum acid phosphatase is a widely used biochemical test to detect prostatic carcinoma. Often the level of the enzyme increases as the disease progresses from intracapsular to extracapsular. Measurement of acid phosphatase is most useful in detecting late stages of the disease. Unfortunately, however, the standard enzymatic determination for serum acid phosphatase has frequently failed to detect intracapsular prostatic carcinoma. Additional assays that will be able to detect intracapsular carcinoma are needed.

A recent study of a radioimmunoassay technique for acid phosphatase shows the radioimmunoassay to be far more sensitive in detecting minimal elevations of acid phosphatase than is the standard biochemical test. The radioimmunoassay diagnosed 33 percent of patients with stage I prostatic carcinoma, compared to only 12 percent diagnosed by the standard assay [3].

The clinical application of the radioimmunoassay as a screening procedure for stage I or II prostatic carcinoma is still uncertain. A larger sample of patients will need to be analyzed to determine an acceptable upper limit of normal. Early data suggest, however, that the radioimmunoassay for prostatic acid phosphatase has the potential to detect over one-half of all cases of intracapsular prostatic carcinoma. In contrast, the enzymatic determination has little or no diagnostic value in detecting intracapsular prostatic carcinoma.

Another promising approach has been the study of lactic dehydrogenase (LDH) isoenzymes from expressed prostatic fluid. The LDH-5/LDH-1 ratio was greater than three in 80 percent of patients with prostatic cancer, compared to 14 percent of patients with benign prostatic hypertrophy and 0 percent of controls [4].

IMMUNOLOGICAL SCREENING

Carcinoembryonic antigens (CEA) have been elevated in 40 to 50 percent of patients with prostatic cancer. Unless greater sensitivity can be obtained, this assay is not clinically useful for early detection.

CYTOLOGY

There is no evidence that exfoliative cytology of either the urine or prostatic fluid is suitable for mass screening [10].

STAGES OF PROSTATIC CARCINOMA

The following are the four stages of prostatic carcinoma:

1. *Stage I*—The tumor is not detectable by rectal examination. The tumor is only detected as a focus of positive microscopic findings from a chip of prostate gland examined, usually after a transurethral resection, for benign prostatic hypertrophy.
2. *Stage II*—The tumor is confined within the prostatic capsule. It may be detectable by rectal examination, and needle biopsy is positive. Bone scan shows no metastasis. There is no lymph node involvement.
3. *Stage III*—The tumor has locally extended beyond the prostatic capsule. Rectal examination and needle biopsy are positive. There is no lymph node involvement, and the bone scan is negative.
4. *Stage IV*—Rectal examination reveals a very hard prostate, and needle biopsy is positive. The bone scan is positive. Other sites may be involved.

Summary and Recommendations

Despite the increasing mortality from carcinoma of the prostate, little is known about its risk factors, etiology, or prevention. Because identification of high-risk groups is not possible, it is most troubling for the primary care physician that no satisfactory method of early detection currently exists. Studies on the natural history of prostatic carcinoma have shown that although many nodules remain quiescent or even regress, many progress from localized and curable carcinoma to regional and metastatic disease with little chance of cure. Early detection must be able to identify those patients with potentially lethal prostatic carcinoma.

Because of the lack of a more suitable screening test, rectal examination and biopsy of suspicious areas remain the only feasible methods of early detection. Rectal examinations, however, will not detect many early prostatic cancers. As a result, at the time of the initial diagnosis, the majority of patients already have far advanced disease.

Although no study has ever shown that frequent rectal examinations will increase the detection of early localized disease, rectal examination remains the first step in diagnosis. Because of the significant percentage of prostatic carcinoma that goes undetected by rectal examination but can be detected by histological examination, it is incumbent upon the primary care physician to insist upon open prostatic biopsy for patients undergoing any urological surgery. Needle aspiration biopsy may provide another useful tool for preliminary office screening of prostatic carcinoma.

References

1. Bauer, W., M. McGavran, and R. Garlin. Unsuspected carcinoma of the prostate in supra-pubic prostatectomy specimens. *Cancer* 13:370, 1960.
2. DeWys, W. Letter to the editor. *N. Engl. J. Med.* 82:428, 1975.
3. Foty, A., et al. Detection of prostatic carcinoma by solid phase radio immuno assay of serum prostatic acid phosphatase. *N. Engl. J. Med.* 297:1357, 1977.
4. Franks, L.M. Etiology, epidemiology and pathology of prostate carcinoma. *Cancer* 32:1092, 1973.

5. Grayhack, J.   Detection of prostatic cancer. *Cancer Chemother. Rep.* 59:139, 1975.

6. Higgins, I.   Epidemiology of carcinoma of the prostate (editorial). *J. Chronic Dis.* 28:343, 1975.

7. Hudson, P., and A. Prout.   Prostatic carcinoma. *N.Y. State J. Med.* 66:351, 1966.

8. Hutchinson, G.   Etiology and prevention of prostatic carcinoma. *Cancer Chemother. Rep.* 59:57, 1975.

9. Jewett, H.   The significance of the palpable prostatic nodule. *J.A.M.A.* 203:403, 1968.

10. Kline, T., et al.   Prostatic carcinoma and a needle aspiration biopsy. *Am. J. Clin. Pathol.* 67:131, 1977.

11. Murphy, G., et al.   Prostatic carcinoma—Treatment at a categorical center 1960–1969. *N.Y. State J. Med.* 75:1663, 1975.

12. Murphy, G.   The diagnosis of prostatic cancer. *Cancer,* 37:689, 1976.

13. Whitmore, W.   The natural history of prostatic cancer. *Cancer* 32:1104, 1973.

14. Wynder, E., K. Mabuchi, and W. Whitmore.   Epidemiology of cancer of the prostate. *Cancer* 28:344, 1971.

8

Motor Vehicle Accidents

Occurrence

Motor vehicle accidents are the leading cause of death for both men and women under age 35 (Fig. 8-1). The automobile is the etiological agent responsible for over fifty-six thousand deaths and four million injuries every year. One out of every two Americans will be involved in an injury-producing collision sometime in his life. Children have a higher mortality from automobile accidents than from the next six leading causes of childhood mortality combined. Automobile accidents are the major killer of young parents. It is strange that in a society that supposedly cares about its children and young adults and that spends great sums of money on the study of other killers, the greatest killer of all, automobile accidents, is virtually ignored.

The clinical interest of physicians concerning motor vehicle accidents has traditionally been in accepting responsibility for the medical and surgical care of accident victims. The orthopedist, the neurosurgeon, and the plastic surgeon are mainly involved. Emergency transportation, intensive care, and rehabilitative programs exist. What is lacking is a commitment by all physicians to apply the skills of prevention to automotive safety. All primary care physicians should be aware of the risk factors asso-

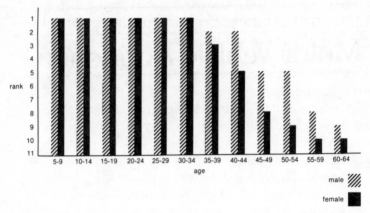

Figure 8-1. *Rank of motor vehicle accidents as cause of death by age.*

ciated with automotive morbidity and mortality and should take appropriate steps to reduce those risks for their patients.

Risk Factors

It is generally agreed that there are three major risk factors associated with a majority of automobile accidents: (1) lack of or improper use of seat belts and child restraints, (2) drinking and driving, and (3) speeds greater than 50 miles per hour. Less important risk factors associated with a minority of accidents include (1) chronic medical conditions of the driver and (2) age and mechanical condition of the car.

SEAT BELTS
The risk of serious or fatal injury is increased by a ratio of 3.35:1 when seat belts are not worn. With the use of lap and shoulder belts, no fatalities occurred in collisions up to 60 miles per hour. It is estimated that up to eighteen thousand fatalities could be avoided each year with the

proper use of seat belts. More recent data suggest that the efficiency of seat belts in decreasing fatalities for all collisions is approximately 50 percent [9]. All new-model cars are now equipped with combination lap and shoulder restraints for front seat occupants and lap belts for rear seat occupants.

The availability of safety belts does not guarantee their use, however. In a 1975 belt-use survey of 5,241 drivers, only 27 percent were using seat belts [8]. The most pressing problem is how motorists can be motivated to use the available restraint systems that can significantly decrease morbidity and mortality in the millions of vehicle collisions that occur annually.

In spite of a number of campaigns urging safety belt use, the proportion of vehicle occupants using belts is so low that much of the decreased morbidity and mortality that could be expected by their use is not being achieved. Public education based upon slogans like "buckle up for safety" and "what's your excuse" had virtually no success. A campaign by the National Safety Council spent the equivalent of $51 million in public service advertising time and space and achieved no increased seat belt usage [10].

In a survey designed to determine which factors corre-lated with the greatest increase in seat belt usage, it was determined that people who had a friend or relative injured, but not killed, in an automobile crash were most likely to use seat belts. In addition, the respondents with more education and those who rated belts most com-fortable and convenient were more likely to use seat belts. At this time, it seems the most successful motivating force to use seat belts that can be utilized by the physician is the fear of disfigurement. It must be noted, however, that a study using a television advertising campaign stress-ing fear of disfigurement and disability still showed no significant increase in seat belt usage.

The role of the primary care physician in increasing seat belt use is unclear at this time [3]. It would seem, however, that the primary care physician is in a key position to increase seat belt use by motivating his patients to use appropriate restraints for themselves and their passengers. Several studies have shown how pediatricians could influence parents to buy and install proper child restraining devices. In a comparison of the effectiveness of face-to-face advice against the effectiveness of two letters, 43 percent of parents receiving the face-to-face advice, versus only 15 percent receiving the letters, installed restraining devices [1]. Another study confirmed that an enthusiastic and persistent physician and his staff could achieve greater than 90-percent parent compliance in obtaining a child restraining device for the family automobile [6].

The failure of motorists to use seat belts may be due in part to the failure of physicians to exercise their influence as effectively as they might. The American Academy of Pediatrics estimates that only 58 percent of pediatricians ever discuss car safety with parents. Only 3 percent advise parents about car safety during each visit. In a study aimed at increasing the teaching behavior of physicians in regard to automotive safety, pediatricians either received a mailed questionnaire from the local chapter of the American Academy of Pediatrics or were given a brief presentation by a local pharmaceutical representative [6]. In a 1-month follow-up, 61 percent of the mailing group and 49 percent of the interview group claimed that their teaching on this subject had increased. Although it has been demonstrated that pediatricians can be influenced to increase their teaching on the subject of automotive safety, the long-term effect of this teaching on altering behavior is unclear.

Although there exists no known means of achieving universal seat belt use, several techniques have, temporarily at least, increased usage. The ignition interlock systems present on 1974-model cars increased use to 60 percent.

By late 1974, however, the ignition interlock was banned as federally required equipment on new cars.

Mandatory belt-use laws in Victoria, Australia have increased belt use to 75 percent, with a subsequent decrease of automobile fatalities by 21 percent. Despite the success of such a law in reducing automobile fatalities, no such mandatory law has yet been passed by any state in this country.

Passive restraint systems, such as automatic seat belts and air bags, are already saving lives. The fatality rate for cars with automatic seat belts was 0.78 deaths per 100 million miles, compared to 2.34 deaths per 100 million miles for similar cars equipped with standard belts. After 600 million miles of travel by cars equipped with air bags, the fatality rate was 0.85 deaths per 100 million miles, about one-half the rate observed in similar cars equipped with manual belts.

Federal regulations require that passive automobile restraints be installed in 1982-model full-sized cars, in 1983 intermediate-sized cars, and in 1984 compact and subcompact cars.

Car Safety Restraints for Children. The prenatal period seems to be an ideal time to counsel parents in car safety because

1. Prospective parents are relatively free of immediate demands and have time to act on recommendations.
2. Prospective parents are eagerly planning for the new baby and are motivated to "do the right thing."
3. Baby gifts are a common means of obtaining an infant car seat.

In a study of the effectiveness of car safety counseling during the prenatal period, 69 percent of the counseled, versus only 42 percent of the noncounseled mothers, were using a safe infant restraint system at the 6-week visit [5].

Infants and children require special car restraints. Small children must be protected by distributing the force of a collision over a large body area. Special restraints should be used until a child weighs at least 18.1 kg (40 lb). If no special device is available, standard seat belts are preferable to no restraint [11]. However, the use of standard belts with children presents the following problems:

1. In an adult, the prominent anterior superior iliac spines are used as anchor points. In a child, these are not well developed until after 10 years of age.
2. The increased bulges of flesh in the pelvic region of a child make correct positioning of a lap belt difficult. The belt could subsequently ride up, causing intra-abdominal injuries in a collision.
3. A small child's higher center of gravity, resulting in a greater body mass above the belt, may cause the child to whip forward in a collision more than an adult would.

Although admittedly data are limited, until better data are available the following conclusions can be drawn in regard to child restraints [12]:

1. Children under 6 years old and infants should wear specially designed child or infant restraining devices.
2. Lap belt restraints appear to offer protection even for younger children. Where proper child restraints are not available, parents should utilize lap belts as a second choice.
3. The preponderance of evidence suggests that any occupant— infant, child, or adult—is far less likely to be killed or injured in a crash while restrained. Combination lap and shoulder belts, although designed for adults, can be used for small children when a child restraining device is not available. In some cases, where the shoulder belt obviously does not fit, it may be necessary to place the shoulder component behind the child, using only the lap belt for restraint.
4. Child seats that hook over regular automobile seats should not be used.
5. Under no circumstances should children or infants be unrestrained in a motor vehicle.

Consumers Union, a nonprofit consumer testing service, tested 14 commonly available models of child restraining devices. In addition to testing the devices in simulated crash tests, other factors such as convenience were checked. The more awkward or more time-consuming it was to seat the child, the less likely the restraint was to be used properly, if at all. The five top-rated child safety restraints are

1. Strolle Wee Care Car Seat 597S
2. Century Motor-Toter
3. GM Child Love Seat
4. Swyngomatic American Safety Seat 300
5. Teddy Tot Astroseat V

These top-rated models all require installation, according to the manufacturer's directions, with a tether. A front seat tether is not a serious inconvenience. A rear seat tether, however, involves installing a permanent anchor for it. In any event, proper installation and use of a restraining device is essential for maximum protection.

Safety experts recommend placing the child restraining device in the center of the rear seat (in cars that have a belt in the center rear position). In a crash, the back of most front seats has a softer, less dangerous surface than does the rigid dashboard. The firmness of the center area of a rear bench seat minimizes the child's head movement in a crash. When the restraining device is equidistant from each side of the car, the child is less likely to slam against the interior if the car is struck from the side.

Further useful information, including handout literature and a film on car safety for children, can be obtained from the Physicians for Automotive Safety, Irvington, New Jersey.

DRINKING
The relationship between alcohol use and abuse, alcoholism, and highway safety is complex. Although it is clear that the combination of alcohol and driving is dangerous,

many variables are involved in each situation, including the driver's blood alcohol level, his previous experience with both drinking and driving, traffic density, and speed.

Of the fourteen million motor vehicle accidents occurring annually, at least eight hundred thousand are alcohol related. Approximately one-half of all highway deaths are alcohol related. Alcohol is the single most prevalent factor in multiple vehicle accidents, in single vehicle accidents, and in accidents involving pedestrians.

Although alcohol affects all cells of the body, the most dramatic effect occurs upon the central nervous system. Driving skill begins to deteriorate at blood alcohol levels below 0.05 percent. This level is reached in a 190-pound person who consumes three 12-ounce beers or three drinks containing 1 ounce of 86-proof alcohol within 1 hour of driving. A 120-pound person can achieve the same blood alcohol level with fewer than two beers or fewer than two 1-ounce drinks. The ingestion of food and the rate of consumption may also influence blood alcohol levels.

Increasing concentrations of alcohol in the blood are well correlated with increased automobile accidents. Blood alcohol levels of 0.05 percent produce carelessness, decreased exactitude in braking and in steering, and a greater tendency to drive toward the edge of the road. With 0.1 percent blood alcohol levels, drivers consistently fluctuate between low and high speeds, swerve from lane to lane, and use excessive time to return to the correct lane.

It has been customary to blame many alcohol-related accidents on the "social" drinker. Many recent studies have demonstrated, however, that a large proportion of drinking drivers have serious alcohol problems [4]. In one study, 70.6 percent of people arrested for driving while intoxicated had blood alcohol levels greater than 115 mg/100 ml, and 36.2 percent had blood alcohol levels greater than 200 mg/100 ml. In order for a 160-pound man to achieve a blood alcohol level of 200 mg/100 ml, he would have to consume eight 12-ounce bottles of beer or 12 ounces of 80-proof liquor on an empty stomach within 1 hour. Significantly, only 3.9 percent of those arrested for driving while intoxicated ever received any kind of treatment for their alcohol problem. Despite their arrest, 90 percent considered their drinking not to be a problem. Clearly, this population is in desperate need of intensive treatment to prevent further dependency upon alcohol (see Chap. 9 for a discussion on alcohol treatment).

SPEEDS OVER 50 MILES PER HOUR

The risk of serious or fatal injury increases by a ratio of 4.87 : 1 with speeds over 50 miles per hour [7]. The reduction in 1974 of the national speed limit to 55 miles per hour is generally credited with significantly reducing highway morbidity and mortality. The death rate from motor vehicle accidents decreased 17 percent from 1973 to 1974 and an additional 5 percent in 1975 (Fig. 8-2). The 1975 death rate is the lowest since 1943 and 1944 when restrictions resulting from World War II severely limited the use of the automobile.

MINOR RISK FACTORS

Chronic medical conditions of the driver and mechanical failure of the car are responsible for a minority of fatalities. The driving records of 2,672 people with chronic medical conditions were compared to the driving records of a control group [13]. Drivers with diabetes mellitus, epilepsy, cardiovascular disease, or mental illness averaged twice the accident rate per 100,000 miles of driving as the controls. The risk increased for drivers with chronic conditions who were over the age of 60, for those with a poor attitude toward driving and toward maintaining a proper medical regime, for those with severe illnesses, and for those with a past history of an accident related to their medical condition.

The mechanical condition of the car is a small contributor to fatality. In a study comparing death rates from

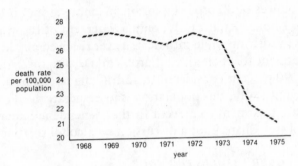

Figure 8-2. *Death rate by year from motor vehicle accidents.*

automobile accidents in states with inspection programs to death rates in states without inspection programs, a clear association was established between the procedure of inspection and a decrease in the death rate [2]. Older cars are more likely than newer cars to be involved in an accident. The likelihood of a fatal accident occurring in a car less than 2 years old is relatively low. The risk increases with the age of the car, doubling for a car greater than 8 years old.

Summary and Recommendations

The primary care physician can contribute to decreasing the alarmingly high morbidity and mortality from motor vehicle accidents by incorporating automotive safety counseling into routine health services. Lack of seat belt use, drinking with driving, and excess speeds are associated with a majority of accidents.

Several studies have already shown that the primary care physician can significantly reduce automotive morbidity and mortality by motivating patients to use proper restraining devices. Prescription blanks "ordering" the use of car safety procedures, such as proper child restraints or the proper use of seat belts, could supplement periodic discussions about auto safety. The prenatal period is an ideal time to start automobile safety counseling for prospective parents regarding their infants. Periodic reinforcement at subsequent visits achieves even greater compliance. Although few studies have been done with adults, it is likely that constant reinforcement by the primary physician could also achieve significant improvement in seat belt use.

Reduction of the other two major risk factors, alcohol and excess speeds, would be highly desirable. Because no studies have yet examined the role of the primary care physician in reducing these risk factors, no recommendations or guidelines exist. Nevertheless, it seems that the primary care physician is in an ideal position to at least counsel his patients. The more aggressive physicians may even be willing to limit driving privileges for patients with chronic alcohol problems, much as they already do for patients with chronic medical conditions.

RECOMMENDATIONS

1. Automotive safety counseling should be incorporated into general preventive health programs. The earlier started and the more frequently done, the better.
2. Primary care physicians should educate patients about the risk of drinking and driving. They also should consider recommending that known alcohol abusers limit their driving.
3. Primary care physicians should educate patients about the increasing risk of fatal injury with increasing speeds.
4. Primary care physicians should consider recommending that patients with severe chronic medical conditions who are over the age of 60, or who have a poor attitude or a poor driving record, limit their driving.

References

1. Bass, L., and T. Wilson. The pediatrician's influence in private practice measured by a controlled seat belt study. *Pediatrics* 33:700, 1964.

2. Buxbaum, R., and T. Culton. Relationship of motor vehicle inspections to accident mortality. *J.A.M.A.* 197:101, 1966.
3. Charles, S., and J. States. Physician responsibility in prevention of bodily injuries by the automobile. *J.A.M.A.* 197:107, 1966.
4. Fine, E., and P. Scoles. Secondary prevention of alcoholism using population of offenders arrested for driving while intoxicated. *Ann. N.Y. Acad. Sci.* 273:637, 1976.
5. Kanthor, H. Car safety for infants: Effectiveness of prenatal counselling. *Pediatrics* 58(3):320, 1976.
6. Lieberman, H., W. Emmet, and A. Colson. Pediatric automotive restraints, pediatricians and the academy. *Pediatrics* 58(3):316, 1976.
7. McCarroll, J., and W. Haddon. A controlled study of fatal automobile accidents in New York City. *J. Chronic Dis.* 15:811, 1962.
8. Pyle, H. Safety belts: The real preventive medicine in automotive safety. *Prev. Med.* 2:3, 1973.
9. Robertson, L. Estimates of motor vehicle seat belt effectiveness and use: Implications for occupant crash protection. *Am. J. Public Health* 66(9):859, 1976.
10. Robertson, L., et al. A controlled study of the effect of TV messages on safety belt use. *Am. J. Public Health* 64:1071, 1974.
11. Shelness, A.M., and S. Charles. Children as passengers in automobiles: The neglected minority on the nation's highways. *Pediatrics* 56(2):271, 1975.
12. Snyder, R. Are automotive belt systems hazardous to children? *Am. J. Dis. Child.* 129:946, 1975.
13. Waller, J. Chronic medical conditions and traffic safety. *N. Engl. J. Med.* 273:1413, 1965.

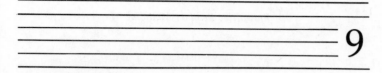

9

Cirrhosis

Occurrence

Mortality from cirrhosis of the liver has been steadily increasing so that cirrhosis now ranks as the seventh leading cause of death in the United States (Fig. 9-1). The death rate from cirrhosis doubled from 7.7 deaths per 100,000 in 1934 to 15.8 deaths per 100,000 in 1974. During one 10-year period, the death rate increased by a sharp 25 percent from 12.1 deaths per 100,000 in 1964 to 15.1 deaths per 100,000 in 1975.

A significant association exists between changes in the death rate from cirrhosis and changes in the consumption of alcoholic beverages [14]. From 1900 to 1914, the death rate varied between 13 and 15 deaths per 100,000. From 1916 through 1920, the death rate decreased to a low of 7 deaths per 100,000, corresponding with the period of effective wartime prohibition. The low rate continued through 1933 while prohibition was in effect. Since the repeal of prohibition in 1933, there has been a steady increase in the cirrhosis death rate corresponding with an increase in per capita consumption of alcoholic beverages.

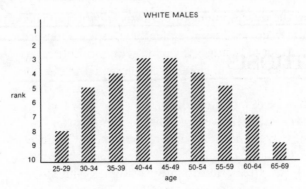

Figure 9-1. *Rank of cirrhosis as cause of death by age.*

Etiology

To clarify the etiology of cirrhosis, in 1974 the International Association for the Study of the Liver adopted a revised etiological classification of cirrhosis [5] :

1. Cirrhosis of genetic disorders—galactosemia glycogen storage diseases, tyrosinosis, hereditary fructose intolerance, $alpha_1$-antitrypsin deficiency, thalassemia, Wilson's disease, hemochromatosis, mucoviscidosis, others
2. Chemical cirrhosis
3. Alcoholic cirrhosis
4. Infections—following viral hepatitis type B, congenital syphilis
5. Nutritional deficiencies
6. Secondary biliary cirrhosis
7. Congestive cirrhosis
8. Primary biliary cirrhosis
9. Cryptogenic cirrhosis—no known etiology
10. Indian childhood cirrhosis
11. Sarcoid

Although chemical toxins, infections, nutritional deficiencies, and diseases of the bile ducts are often contributing factors in the development of cirrhosis, alcoholism is considered the major contributing factor. Despite widespread underreporting of deaths associated with alcoholism, one-third of all deaths from cirrhosis are certified as due to alcohol [11]. In fact, a far larger proportion of cirrhosis deaths may be due to alcoholism.

The relationship between alcohol and cirrhosis is the subject of current debate. Since not all alcoholics develop cirrhosis, alcohol by itself may not be sufficient to produce cirrhosis. In a series of autopsy studies, only 24 to 28 percent of alcoholics had cirrhosis. In a more recent series using liver biopsies, the incidence of cirrhosis among alcoholics was 30 percent [8]. Although specific predisposing biological factors are not known, possible contributing factors are the dosage of alcohol intake, the length of time during which the intake is maintained, and immunological susceptibility. In a study of 526 male alcoholics, it was demonstrated that a close correlation existed between incidence of cirrhosis and the total volume of alcohol ingested [9]. In addition to the time-dose factors, the risk of cirrhosis may ultimately be determined by individual susceptibility.

Alcoholic liver disease may progress from fatty liver to alcoholic hepatitis to cirrhosis [9]. Up to 90 percent of chronic alcoholics have fatty liver, an accumulation of excess fat in the liver. This stage of alcoholic liver disease is benign and fully reversible. However, a more severe form of alcoholic injury, alcoholic hepatitis, may follow when large numbers of cells die, causing necrosis and inflammation. In contrast to the benign and reversible fatty metamorphosis, 80 percent of patients with alcoholic hepatitis who continue to drink develop cirrhosis. Unfortunately, in some patients, possibly because of altered immune mechanisms caused by alcoholic hepatitis, the condition will also progress to cirrhosis despite a discontinuance of alcohol [7]. Alcoholic hepatitis, because of its propensity to lead to cirrhosis and because of its potential reversibility, becomes the critical lesion to identify and treat in the alcoholic patient.

Alcoholism, alcoholic dependence, or *alcohol addiction* describes a condition in which the individual has lost control over his drinking and is unable to abstain. The essential features of the alcohol-dependent states are [3]

1. A subjective awareness that "drink has become a drug."
2. Withdrawal phenomena—Since alcohol is a short-acting drug, withdrawal symptoms appear a few hours after abstinence. For example, morning withdrawal may be manifested by shakes, sweating, or butterflies in the stomach.
3. Tolerance—At first there is a raised tolerance, then in later stages tolerance decreases so that the alcoholic "gets drunk" on less.
4. Amnesias—Although there may be no actual loss of consciousness and the alcoholic can continue to perform complicated tasks such as driving, the morning after he often cannot remember what he did while drunk.

Alcoholism has been formally and scientifically recognized as a disease by the American College of Physicians, the American Medical Association, the American Psychiatric Association, and the World Health Organization. Alcoholism is a chronic, progressive disease that may interfere with health and social and economic functioning. The Department of Health, Education, and Welfare has declared alcoholism to be "the Nation's number 1 health problem." It is a major cause of disrupted family life, automobile and industrial accidents, poor job performance, and increasing crime rates.

Of all fatal automobile accidents, 50 percent involve alcohol. Fifty-three percent of fire deaths, 45 percent of drownings, 22 percent of home accidents, and 36 percent of pedestrian accidents are linked to alcohol abuse. Between 6 and 10 percent of all employees are alcoholics, resulting in over $25 billion per year lost from absenteeism, accidents, and medical expenses. Violent crimes attributed to alcohol abuse account for 64 percent of murders, 41 percent of assaults, 34 percent of rapes, 30 percent of suicides, and 60 percent of child abuse.*

Although alcoholism is the major etiological factor in cirrhosis, the precise etiology of alcoholism itself is unclear. Most authorities agree that there is no single cause of alcoholism. Rather, multiple physiological, psychological, and sociological factors lead to the onset and development of alcoholism.

Although little is currently known about the physiological factors that may contribute to the etiology of alcoholism, some proposed hypotheses include a predisposing biological dysfunction that alters sensitivity to alcohol, a preexisting psychoendocrine disorder, nutritional disorders, and the imbalance of acetylcholine at receptor sites in the ascending reticular formation of the brain stem.

Psychological factors certainly contribute to the etiology of alcoholism. However, it is difficult to determine which psychological traits are causal and which are the results of the illness. The psychoanalytic approach generally holds that alcoholism is the result of early emotional disturbance and deprivation. Emotional immaturity, the underlying personality pattern of alcoholics, leads the alcoholic to rely on the effects of alcohol to relieve feelings of anxiety, hostility, and depression. These feelings may, in fact, represent unrecognized patterns of insecurity, rage, and guilt. The severity of alcoholism is thought to depend upon the level of psychological adjustment just prior to the start of the illness.

Alternatively, learning theorists see alcoholism as a learned behavior. Since ingestion of alcohol may provide an emotional reward, such as reduction of anxiety, more rapidly than other behavior does, it provides reinforcement each time it is used for that purpose. The condi-

---

*Statistics supplied by the National Council on Alcoholism.

tioned response becomes strengthened and may establish drinking as the predominant response to many life situations.

Although no sociological factor can be identified as having uniquely causative effects, such factors as attitudes toward alcohol and the standards applied to the use of alcohol by different groups in society are of great importance in the origin and development of alcoholism.

Risk Factors

A national survey of American drinking practices revealed that drinking is a common behavior [2]. Only 32 percent of adults are abstainers (Table 9-1).

Heavy drinks are likely to be male and are usually younger and live in more urbanized areas than lighter drinkers. They report more drinking by parents and friends, find good things to say about drinking, and find drinking helpful in relieving depression.

SEX

A higher proportion of men (77%) than women (60%) are drinkers. Almost four times as many men as women are heavy drinkers.

AGE

The incidence of drinking and the extent of heavy drinking decrease with age. There is a peak of heavy drinking between ages 45 and 49 and a secondary peak between ages 21 and 24. Forty percent of male drinkers between 45 and 49 years of age are heavy drinkers, compared to only 11 percent of male drinkers over age 65 (Fig. 9-2). The decline of heavy drinking in older age groups may be related to changed metabolism (older people may have more unpleasant physical reactions to alcohol) or to a changed psychology (less tension or alternate modes of coping with stress) or to changed life-cycle phenomena.

Table 9-1. National Drinking Practices

Drinking Classification	Drinking Frequency	Percentage
Abstainers	Less than once per year	32%
Infrequent drinkers	At least once per year, less than once per month	15%
Light drinkers	At least once per month, typically one or two drinks on single occasions	28%
Moderate drinkers	At least once per month, typically several times, usually no more than three or four drinks per occasion	13%
Heavy drinkers	Nearly every day, with five or more drinks per occasion at least once in a while	12%

Source: Adapted from D. Cahalan, I.H. Cisin, and H.M. Crossley. *American Drinking Practices: A National Study of Drinking Behavior and Attitudes.* (Monographs of the Rutgers Center of Alcohol Studies, No. 6.) 1969. Copyright by Journal of Studies on Alcohol, Inc., New Brunswick, N.J. 08903. Reprinted by permission from Journal of Studies on Alcohol, Inc.

SOCIAL STATUS

Those in the higher social classes are more likely to be drinkers but less likely to be heavy drinkers than are those of lower social classes. Using income alone as a measure of social position, in families with incomes under $2,000 per year, 44 percent of persons drink at least once a year. In families with incomes over $15,000 a year, 84 percent of persons drink at least once a year.

OCCUPATION

The largest proportion of abstainers is in the farm-related group. The largest proportion of heavy drinkers is among semiprofessional and technical workers. Certain occupations, such as working in a brewery or working in the

Preventive Primary Medicine

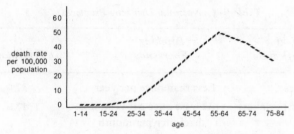

Figure 9-2. *Death rate by age from cirrhosis,*
1975.

catering trade, have far higher proportions of heavy
drinkers.

MARITAL STATUS

There are higher proportions of heavy drinkers among
single, divorced, and separated individuals than among
married and widowed people. Although a causal relationship cannot be established, it is likely that divorced and
separated people are less well adjusted and therefore drink
more.

FAMILY HISTORY

One study reports that a child or sibling of an alcoholic
has 12 times more risk of becoming an alcoholic than does
a child from a nonalcoholic family.

ETHNICITY

Several studies have shown differences in drinking habits
of various ethnic groups. In most cases, in ethnic groups
where alcoholic beverages of low concentration, such as
wine and beer, are available on an everyday basis to all
family members, the rate of alcoholism appears to be
lower than in groups where alcohol is consumed less routinely and more as a means of escape.

ESCAPE DRINKING

Heavy drinking alone is not as likely to lead to alcohol-
related problems as is heavy drinking coupled with non-

socially oriented reasons for drinking. One-half of heavy drinkers can be further classified as heavy escape drinkers in that they drink to escape problems of everyday living. Although heavy escape drinkers are not necessarily alcoholics, since many have no other alcohol-related problems, this group includes many, if not most, alcoholics. The escape drinker is more unhappy with his progress in life, is more likely to exhibit neurotic tendencies, and is more dependent upon external aids to alleviate depression or neurosis. The escape drinker is more likely to mass his drinks on a single occasion. This type of drinker has more alcohol-related problems than drinkers of the same overall volume who space their drinks over more occasions.

Screening and Early Detection

Although excessive drinking is not a rare condition, the recognition of problem drinkers is difficult. It is estimated that 90 percent of patients with drinking problems go undiagnosed by their primary care physician [3]. In an average general practice of 3,000 patients, 6 will be suffering severe physical consequences of alcoholism, and 24 more will be alcoholics or well on their way toward alcoholism. Typically, in only 3 of the 30 patients will the problem be recognized.

The recognition of alcoholism in its early stages is difficult because of the characteristic denial mechanisms used by the alcoholic. The patient with an alcohol-related problem will not often voluntarily seek help from his family doctor. Because the typical physician often finds that dealing with alcoholism can be unrewarding, frustrating, and often hopeless, the average physician has not been aggressive in seeking out the signs of early alcoholism. In order for the primary care physician to be able to recognize alcohol-related problems early in their course, it is essential that a high index of suspicion, coupled with a

positive search for possible signs and symptoms, be
maintained.

SCREENING TESTS

Several attempts have been made to develop clinically
useful screening tests. The British have developed an Alcoholic At Risk Register encompassing nine major risk
factors [16]. According to this screening test, there is a
100-percent probability of a patient's being an alcoholic
if the patient previously asked for help to treat his drinking. There is a 75-percent probability of alcoholism if the
patient smelled of alcohol during an office visit. There is a
50-percent probability of alcoholism if the patient had
symptoms of peptic ulcer or gastritis or requested a sick
note for symptoms that did not appear genuine. There is
a 25-percent probability of alcoholism if the patient pre-
sented with anxiety or depression, worked in a brewery or
catering trade, was divorced or separated or had a history
of marital disharmony, or was a single man over 40 years
old.

The Michigan Alcoholism Screening Test (MAST) makes
use of the observation that a report of excessive drinking
is the best indicator of risk [12, 17]. Although the MAST
has been widely used and has proved effective in detecting
early alcoholism among inpatients, one study revealed
that the MAST could also be adapted to the outpatient
setting [1]. A self-administered, 24-item questionnaire
was given to 252 patients attending a general medical
clinic. In 17 percent of patients, the MAST was the only
readily available means by which alcoholism could be
suspected. A 10-percent incidence of false negatives, presumably due to deliberate covering up, detracts only
slightly from its utility.

The 24 items of the MAST appear in Table 9-2. A score
of 4 is suspicious of alcoholism, and a score of 5 or more
is presumptive. Even though the original 24 items take
less than 5 minutes to complete, they have been condensed

into a 10-item questionnaire. This condensed version, however, has not been adequately tested to recommend its use [12].

BEHAVIORAL CHARACTERISTICS

Even in its early stages, alcoholism may be definable by behavioral characteristics affecting the individual's lifestyle. Alcoholics are typically depressed, tense, self-centered, hypochrondriacal, impulsive, immature, and hostile. Aggression is frequently associated with alcoholism and may be manifested by frequent fighting and violent crimes. A high proportion of automobile accidents involve alcohol in both pedestrians and drivers. At work, alcoholism has a negative effect upon performance and often leads to frequent changes of jobs. Social relationships with family and friends become strained and often broken. Sexual impotence and paranoia are frequent and further impair interpersonal, particularly marital, relationships. Many alcoholics become depressed, and suicide attempts are not uncommon. Although the incidence of suicide attempts among an alcoholic population is not known, among completed suicides alcoholism is an important factor.

PHYSICAL SIGNS

Just as the alcoholic patient will often not conform to the skid-row stereotype, the alcoholic patient will often not have gross physical signs of alcoholism. Changes in speech, facial appearance, and skin may provide the astute primary care physician with the first clinical indication of hidden heavy drinking [5, 13]. Alcohol produces edema of the vocal cords, nasal mucosa, larynx, and posterior pharynx, which may give some alcoholics a characteristic hoarse voice. In early alcoholism, the skin and subcutaneous tissues of the face are puffy and edematous. Later, subcutaneous fat is lost, and the dermis atrophies. Conjunctival vessels may become engorged, along with a general

Table 9-2. *The Michigan Alcoholism Screening Test, Self-administered Version*

MAST Questions	Score	Positive Answer
1. Do you feel you are a normal drinker? (By normal we mean you drink less than or as much as most other people.)	2	No
2. Have you ever awakened the morning after some drinking the night before and found that you could not remember a part of the evening before?	2	Yes
3. Does your wife, husband, a parent, or other near relative ever worry or complain about your drinking?	1	Yes
4. Can you stop drinking without a struggle after one or two drinks?	2	No
5. Do you ever feel guilty about your drinking?	1	Yes
6. Do your friends or relatives think you are a normal drinker?	2	No
7. Are you always able to stop drinking when you want to?	2	No
8. Have you ever attended a meeting of Alcoholics Anonymous (AA) for yourself?	5	Yes
9. Have you gotten into fights when drinking?	1	Yes
10. Has drinking ever created problems between you and your wife, husband, a parent, or other near relative?	2	Yes
11. Has your wife, husband, parent, or other near relative ever gone to anyone for help about your drinking?	2	Yes

12. Have you ever lost friends or girlfriends/boyfriends because of drinking?   2   Yes
13. Have you ever gotten into trouble at work because of drinking?   2   Yes
14. Have you ever lost a job because of drinking?   2   Yes
15. Have you ever neglected your obligations, your family or your work for more than two days in a row because you were drinking?   2   Yes
16. Do you drink before noon fairly often?   1   Yes
17. Have you ever been told you have liver trouble? Cirrhosis?   2   Yes
18. Have you ever had delirium (DTs), severe shaking, heard voices, or seen things that weren't there after heavy drinking?   5   Yes
19. Have you ever gone to anyone for help about your drinking?   5   Yes
20. Have you ever been in a hospital because of drinking?   5   Yes
21. Have you ever been a patient in a psychiatric hospital or on a psychiatric ward of a general hospital where drinking was part of the problem?   2   Yes
22. Have you ever been seen at a psychiatric or mental health clinic, or gone to a doctor, social worker, or clergyman for help with an emotional problem in which drinking had played a part?   2   Yes
23. Have you ever been arrested, even for a few hours, because of drunk behavior?   2   Yes
24. Have you ever been arrested for drunken driving, driving while intoxicated, or driving under the influence of alcoholic beverage?   2   Yes

Scoring: 4 = suspicious of alcoholism; 5 or more = presumptive of alcoholism.
Source: Breitenbucher [1].

dilatation of the facial vessels, causing a flushed appearance not to be confused with rosacea. Cigarette burns on the hands or chest or nicotine stains on the fingers or repeated ecchymoses, abrasions, or lacerations, particularly on the shins, knees, face, or head, from repeated falls provide discernible clues.

Other nonspecific lesions occurring in association with alcoholism are pronounced ecchymoses at the site of venipuncture (perhaps secondary to an alcohol-related bleeding disorder), fungal infections of the nails, slow-healing abrasions, and a form of melanosis manifested as a dirty tan hue most pronounced on sun-exposed areas. Vascular spiders, palmar erythema, and corkscrew scleral vessels reflect advanced liver disease.

Hepatomegaly will not be found as often as will subtle hepatic tenderness. Alcoholic neuritis is uncommon compared to the frequency of absent or diminished ankle jerks. An obvious tremor is unlikely, but a slight tremor of the hands or tongue is more likely, as are mild signs of avitaminosis.

Prevention

PRIMARY PREVENTION

In contrast to the increasing death rate from cirrhosis in the United States, the death rate from cirrhosis in Great Britain has been decreasing. In 1914, the death rate from cirrhosis in Great Britain was 10 deaths per 100,000, which fell to 5 deaths per 100,000 in 1920, then gradually decreased to a low of 2 deaths per 100,000 in the 1940s, and rose only to a rate of 3 deaths per 100,000 in 1963. The British succeeded in lowering their cirrhosis death rate by 70 percent because of their social policy on alcoholic beverages. Since cirrhosis mortality is directly related to the per capita consumption of alcohol, prevention must be linked with lowering that consumption. After World War I, when restrictions on the amount of alcoholic beverages sold were removed, the government progressively increased the taxes and severely limited the hours of sale of alcoholic beverages. Per capita consumption decreased from 0.59 gallons in 1913 to 0.25 gallons in 1936.

Despite the success of the British in lowering the cirrhosis death rate by reducing per capita consumption, progressive taxation and regulation are unlikely alternatives in this country for the foreseeable future. Indeed, alcoholism and alcohol abuse have only recently become recognized as serious health and social problems. In the 1974 Comprehensive Alcohol Abuse and Alcoholics Prevention, Treatment and Rehabilitation Act, Congress found that

1. *Alcohol is one of the most dangerous drugs and the drug most frequently abused in the United States;*
2. *Of the nation's estimated 95 million drinkers, at least 9 million, or 7% of the adult population, are alcohol abusers and alcoholics;*
3. *Problem drinking costs the national economy at least fifteen billion dollars annually in lost working time, medical and public assistance expenditures, and police and court costs;*
4. *Alcohol abusers are found with increasing frequency among persons who are multiple drug abusers and among former heroin addicts who are being treated in methadone maintenance programs;*
5. *Alcohol abuse is being discovered among growing numbers of youth; and*
6. *Alcoholism is an illness requiring treatment and rehabilitation through the assistance of a broad range of community health and social services, and with the cooperation of law enforcement agencies.*

SECONDARY PREVENTION

Programs to control cirrhosis through early identification and education of alcohol abusers and early treatment and rehabilitation of the alcoholic have achieved some limited success. If the alcohol abuser can be identified, he may be able to be helped. One optimistic author suggested that medical advice is all that is necessary for up to 20 percent of patients with a drinking problem to become permanently sober. Twenty percent will continue to drink, despite the most intensive medical therapy. Of the remaining 60 percent, neither will the majority be immediately helped nor will they immediately reject help [3].

As with many diseases, the sooner treatment is begun, the higher the success rate. In alcoholism, the success of secondary prevention is directly proportional to the time elapsed between the onset of the disease and the time the patient is motivated to accept treatment. In the case of alcoholism, however, unlike many other diseases, the patient often does not want to be treated. Several major problems surrounding early identification and treatment of alcoholism are [15]

1. The difficulty of early detection—In a society that accepts and encourages social drinking, identifying the drinker who exceeds the ill-defined limits of social drinking can be extremely difficult. In addition, the alcoholic is a renowned denier and may possess great skills in concealing his problem.
2. Society's stigmatization of alcoholism—There is a powerful incentive to conceal the disease as long as society views alcohol abuse as a "self-inflicted disease" brought on by irresponsible, morally weak individuals.
3. Power of the addiction—Alcohol is such a powerful addictor that often the victim does not believe he can live without alcohol. Living without alcohol may indeed be so terrifying that motivation for concealment of the problem is even further reinforced.
4. The guilt and shame of the victim—The victim has a feeling of guilt and shame, which may prevent him from admitting his problem and seeking treatment.

The National Council on Alcoholism has developed a very successful approach to the early detection of the employed alcoholic. After extensive surveys of employee absenteeism records, it became clear that every employee suffering from alcoholism, even in its early stages, demonstrates a readily observable deteriorating pattern of job performance. This pattern of deteriorating job performance is manifested through such objective factors as absenteeism, poor judgment, erratic performance, decreasing productivity, lateness and early departures, customer complaints, failure to meet deadlines, and other evidence of poor performance.

Employees whose job performance drops below acceptable standards may be referred to a professional counseling and diagnostic service for identification and appropriate treatment of the problem. At least during the early stages of alcoholism, the employee often still has a strong desire to hold onto his job. The clear-cut choice between accepting assistance and accepting the regular disciplinary consequences of poor job performance is a powerful motivating force encouraging employees to accept treatment.

This approach of monitoring job performance and offering assistance to those who need it results in alcoholism recovery rates ranging from 60 to 80 percent. Unfortunately, of the 1.6 million American corporations, only three to four hundred have any type of alcohol rehabilitation program.

The role of the primary care physician can be most influential in treating alcoholics. Many primary care physicians, unfortunately, do not play as essential a role in the early identification and continual treatment of the alcoholic as might be possible. In a recent poll, although 90 percent of physicians sampled had at some previous time treated an alcoholic, only 45 percent indicated any continuing contact with an alcoholic patient [6].

Four factors have contributed to physicians' reluctance to treat alcohol-related problems:

1. The moral attitude of physicians—The moral attitude and perceptions of certain physicians may influence their approach to alcoholism. Of sampled physicians, 25 percent believed moral weakness was the main determinant of alcoholism. A

study of family practice residents revealed that they rated alcoholics as weaker, more helpless, and more aimless than average
persons [4]. This negative attitude, similar to society's stigmatization of alcoholism, may contribute to the lack of vigorous
screening attempts and adequate early treatment by primary
care physicians.

2. Lack of adequate exposure to the full spectrum of alcoholic
   patients—Few medical schools or residency training programs
   offer training in alcoholism treatment and prevention. The only
   contact most physicians in training have with the alcoholic
   patient is in the emergency room or in the intensive care unit,
   where they are confronted with the far-advanced, life-endanger-
   ing medical complications of alcoholism. Rarely have these
   physicians the opportunity to treat alcoholic patients early in
   the course of their disease. It has been demonstrated, however,
   that the more contact a physician has with alcoholics, the more
   positive his attitude becomes. Perhaps by increasing exposure
   to the alcoholic patient in medical school and residency training
   and by dispelling the notion that medical treatment of alcoholism is frustrating and useless, a more realistic approach to
   identifying and treating the major cause of cirrhosis can be
   developed.

3. Lack of continual, family-oriented, and coordinated care—
   Continual, family-oriented, and coordinated care can improve
   early treatment of the alcoholic. The patient with an alcohol-
   related problem requires the assistance, support, and trust of
   the physician that is built up through continual care. Successful
   treatment also requires evaluation of the entire family and the
   patient's social situation. It is usually impossible to help an
   alcoholic without also knowing the spouse and other family
   members and without understanding how their behavior contributed to the drinking problem. It is also essential to know
   something about the patient's work and leisure habits and their
   support mechanisms. Successful treatment requires integrated
   care. Referral to other treatment sources, such as to a psy-
   chiatrist or Alcoholics Anonymous, is often necessary. The
   primary care physician must be able to coordinate all sources
   of care while maintaining a continual relationship with the
   patient.

4. Lack of early screening for the disease—Newer approaches to
   more aggressive screening for alcoholism, particularly by primary care physicians, are required. Since 1 person in 10 who
   drinks will develop an alcohol-related problem, it is important

to be able to identify those individuals at greater risk. They could then be observed and educated before excessive alcohol abuse occurs.

There may be a subgroup of alcoholics who are subject to very early dependency, within days or weeks of the first time they ever became drunk. Polls show that up to 30 percent of alcoholics believe that this is how they became addicted. If indeed this is true, a means must be developed to identify this very high-risk group so that they can be prevented from ever becoming drunk [10].

Summary and Recommendations

Although cirrhosis may have many etiologies, alcohol is the major contributing factor. The death rate from cirrhosis, which is linked to alcohol consumption, has been steadily increasing in the United States. Drinking is a common practice. One drinker in 10 will develop an alcohol-related problem. This person is likely to be a heavy escape drinker. If he is male, between the ages of 45 and 49, and of lower socioeconomic status, he is at greater risk of becoming an alcoholic.

Early recognition of an alcohol-related problem is difficult. But because of the potential reversibility of early alcoholism, screening and early detection are essential. A high index of suspicion for behavioral characteristics and physical signs can help lead to the recognition of an alcohol problem. To increase sensitivity, the MAST has proved useful in identifying alcohol problems in ambulatory patients.

Limiting the availability of alcohol has proved an effective means of primary prevention. Early identification and treatment of alcohol abusers has also had limited success. The judgmental attitudes of physicians have been detrimental in maximizing their therapeutic impact.

RECOMMENDATIONS

1. The primary care physician should screen for alcohol-related problems by means of the MAST or similar test.
2. The physician should maintain a high index of suspicion for the behavioral and physical signs of alcohol-related problems.
3. Particularly in the high-risk patient, the physician should be alert to requests for "something for nerves" or "something for the stomach." The physician should never prescribe a tranquilizer or antacid without first inquiring about drinking habits.
4. The physician's moral attitude should not interfere with his ability to identify and treat alcoholics. The best way to improve personal perceptions of alcoholics is to work with them.

References

1. Breitenbucher, R. The routine administration of the Michigan Alcoholic Screening Test to ambulatory patients. *Minn. Med.* 59:425, 1976.
2. Cahalan, D., I.H. Cisin, and H.M. Crossley. *American Drinking Practices: A National Study of Drinking Behavior and Attitudes.* Monographs of the Rutgers Center of Alcohol Studies, No. 6. Rutgers Center of Alcohol Studies, New Brunswick, N.J., 1969. Pp. 18–64.
3. Edwards, G. Patients with drinking problems. *Br. Med. J.* 4:435, 1968.
4. Fisher, J., et al. Physicians and alcoholics: Factors affecting attitudes of family practice residents toward alcoholics. *J. Stud. Alcohol* 36:626, 1975.
5. Galambos, J. Classification of cirrhosis. *Am. J. Gastroenterol.* 64:437, 1975.
6. Knott, D., R. Fink, and J. Beard. Unmasking alcohol abuse. *Am. Fam. Physician* 10:123, 1974.
7. Leevy, C., R. Zetterman, and F. Smith. Newer approaches to treatment of liver disease in the alcoholic. *Ann. N.Y. Acad. Sci.* 52:135, 1975.
8. Lelbach, W. Cirrhosis in the alcoholic and its relation to the volume of alcohol abuse. *Ann. N.Y. Acad. Sci.* 252:82, 1975.
9. Lieber, C. Liver disease and alcohol: Fatty liver, alcoholic hepatitis, cirrhosis and their inter-relationships. *Ann. N.Y. Acad. Sci.* 252:63, 1975.
10. Lundberg, G. Susceptibility to dependence on alcohol: Primary and secondary prevention (editorial). *J.A.M.A.* 233:356, 1975.

11. Mortality from cirrhosis of the liver. *Statistical Bulletin of Metropolitan Life Insurance Company* 54:5, October 1973.
12. Pokorny, A., B. Miller, and H. Kaplan. The brief MAST: A shortened version of the Michigan Alcoholism Screening Test. *Am. J. Psychiatry* 129:342, 1972.
13. Silberfarb, P. Recognizing alcoholism early by physical signs. *Postgrad. Med.* 59:79, 1975.
14. Terris, M. Epidemiology of cirrhosis of the liver: National mortality data. *Am. J. Public Health* 57:2076, 1967.
15. Von Wiegand, R. Advantages in secondary prevention of alcoholism through the cooperative efforts of labor and management in employer organizations. *Prev. Med.* 3:80, 1974.
16. Wilkins, R. The hidden alcoholic in general practice. *Br. J. Addict.* (Suppl. 70):12, 1975.
17. Woodruff, R., et al. A brief method for screening alcoholism. *Dis. Nerv. Syst.* 37:434, 1976.

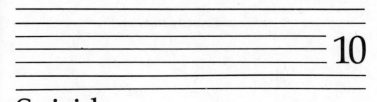

10

Suicide

Occurrence

The suicide rate in the United States has increased steadily over the past 20 years so that suicide is now the tenth leading cause of death among all age groups (Fig. 10-1). The most dramatic increases have occurred in the 15- to 29-year age group. In this age group, suicide is now the second leading cause of death (Fig. 10-2), and the suicide rate among 15- to 29-year-olds is now three times higher than it was just 20 years ago. The even more rapid rise of the attempted suicide rate from 59 cases per 100,000 in 1960 to a currently estimated 730 cases per 100,000 has been referred to as a major epidemic.

Suicidal persons display sufficiently distinct demographic and clinical features to permit their early identification as a high-risk group by the primary care physician. General physicians in Great Britain have taken a lead in early identification and active treatment of these high-risk patients. As a result, the suicide rate is decreasing in Great Britain.

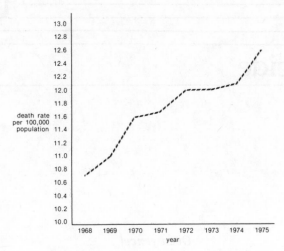

Figure 10-1. Death rate by year from suicide.

Risk Factors for Completed and Attempted Suicide

AGE

The age of peak incidence of successful suicides tends to be in the mid-50s (Fig. 10-3). In a study of 134 suicides in a metropolitan area, 32 percent of successful suicides occurred in the 55- to 65-year age group, 25 percent occurred in the 65- to 75-year age group, and 22 percent occurred in the 45- to 55-year age group [6]. In contrast, suicide attempters tend to be young [3]. There is general agreement that ages 20 to 30, especially 20 to 24, are the peak risk years. Although the average age of attempters has been decreasing over the past decade, 50 percent are under age 30 [3].

SEX

There is an almost equal sex distribution among completed suicides. In contrast, there is a preponderance by 2 : 1 of female to male attempters. The differences in these rates have been attributed to men's using more violent and

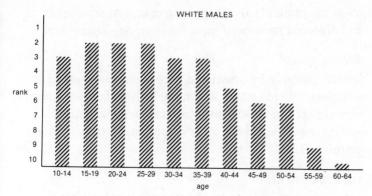

Figure 10-2. *Rank of suicide as cause of death by age.*

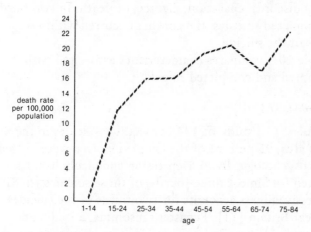

Figure 10-3. *Death rate by age from suicide, 1975.*

effective means, although there is some evidence that male attempters are increasing [12].

MARITAL STATUS
The data for marital status as related to suicide are less clear than for age and sex because separating out confounding variables is difficult. The married state is said to protect against completed suicide, while divorce and widow-

hood facilitate it [6]. There is an excess of separated and divorced persons of both sexes among attempters.

SOCIAL CLASS

Social class may be associated with the seriousness of attempts. Suicide attempts among higher classes are more often judged to be serious, whereas suicide attempts among lower classes are more often judged to be minor gestures [13].

SOCIAL CONFLICT

A suicide or suicide attempt often takes place after a recent serious interpersonal conflict, such as a marital or family discord, separation, divorce, or death. In two-thirds of completed suicides, the conflict occurred within 6 weeks of the suicide.

Table 10-1 compares characteristics associated with attempted and completed suicide.

CLINICAL STATE

Depression. In a study of 134 consecutive suicides in the St. Louis area, 95 percent of the people involved were judged to be psychologically ill. Depression and alcoholism accounted for almost three-fourths of those suicides [6, 8]. Depressive illness accounts for two-thirds of the suicides in Great Britain [11]. Persistent insomnia, a frequent indicator of depression, has often been a symptom associated with suicide. Among suicide attempters, depression is frequently linked to suicidal behavior. Thirty-five to 79 percent of all attempters have been depressed [13]. Further evidence suggests that suicide potential may be related to the severity of the depressive symptoms. In a study of 384 suicide attempters, hopelessness was found to be a key variable linking depression with suicidal behavior [1]. Hopelessness may then be a stronger indicator of suicidal intent than is depression by itself.

Table 10-1. *Attempted Versus Completed Suicide*

Variables	Attempted	Completed
Age	Young	Mid-50s
Sex	Female	Equal
Marital status	Excess separated and divorced	Excess separated and divorced
Depression	35%–79%	68%
Associated physical illness	Rare among hospitalized patients	51%
Alcoholism	Frequently precedes; impulsive act	29%
Social status	After recent interpersonal conflict	After recent interpersonal conflict and social isolation

Alcoholism. Twenty-nine percent of completed suicides are alcoholics. The greater degree of social isolation among alcoholics may predispose this group to a higher suicide rate than the general population. Alcoholics most likely to commit suicide are alcoholics who have suffered a recent loss.

Physical Illness. Early data from the study by Robins and associates of 134 consecutive suicides in St. Louis indicated that only 4 percent of completed suicides had medical illnesses [8]. More recent data from a study of 114 suicide cases in the Seattle area indicate that 70 percent had one or more significant physical illnesses at the time of suicide [6]. Fawcett estimates that physical illnesses contributed to suicide in 51 percent of cases [2]. Rheumatoid arthritis, peptic ulcer, and hypertension had the highest absolute values, while malignancies had the highest ratio of suicide to prevalence of the illness. Urological surgery was also found to precipitate severe depressive episodes in men and often preceded suicide. Chronic hemodialysis also represented an increased risk.

Suicide attempts among hospitalized patients are unusual. In a study of 70,000 admissions at the Peter Bent Brigham Hospital, 17 attempts and no deaths occurred. In a similar study of 20,000 admissions at the Los Angeles County Hospital, 12 attempts and no deaths occurred [7, 10]. All the attempts were impulsive acts associated with increased stress. The attempts were precipitated by loss of emotional support, predominantly by a disruption of relations with medical personnel, less often by conflict with family members. Effective prevention of suicide among hospitalized medical and surgical patients depends upon recognizing high-risk patients, such as those with poor impulse control and those subject to unusual stress, especially the loss of emotional support. Continuity of care and a strong patient–medical staff alliance are important preventive measures.

PREVIOUS ATTEMPTS

People who have made previous suicide attempts represent a high-risk group for subsequent suicide. In a study of 100 suicides, compared to 318 depressed patients, suicide occurred seven times as often among those who had made a previous attempt as among depressed patients [11]. Serious attempters had two to three times the suicide rate of less serious attempters [9].

One of the difficult problems in evaluating a suicide attempt is to define its lethality. Clinicians tend to categorize previous attempts into "serious" and less serious "impulsive gestures." Clinical judgments of relative seriousness generally tend to be subjective. There has been little effort made to quantify factors that are involved in the attempt.

Age, sex, self-reported intent, psychiatric diagnosis, suicidal history, actual inflicted damage, and the particular

method used provide some data for judgment of seriousness. Because of the difference in management (high-risk
patients are usually confined to a hospital, whereas low-
risk patients may be sent home), a less subjective, more
quantifiable way of evaluating the seriousness of suicide attempts is desirable.

One such evaluating method is the Weisman-Worden
"Risk-Rescue" ratio. This approach evaluates the implementation of the suicide attempt as a measure of lethality
[12]. Risk is rated according to the method used and the
actual damage inflicted in a single attempt. Since survival after a suicide attempt may also depend upon the
resources for rescue, rescue factors are also considered.
The ratio of risk to rescue provides a judgment regarding
lethality. From this, the relative seriousness of a given
suicide attempt can be assessed.

While the most important factors in the diagnosis, management, and prognosis of suicidal patients remain the
intent, the implementation, and the resources for post-
attempt correction, an objective scale of lethality will
prove useful. When combined with intent and resources, it
may even provide some predictability of future attempts.
The current use of the risk-rescue ratio, however, is
presently limited to evaluating multiple attempts by the
same individual over a period of time and to comparing
different subjects with respect to their actual attempts.

Prevention

The vast majority of persons who commit suicide had been
under the care of a physician within 6 months of committing suicide. No other person has contact with so great
a proportion of potentially suicidal individuals as does the
physician. All physicians, but primary care physicians in
particular, represent a major opportunity for suicide
prevention. The primary care physician has a special ad-

vantage in early case finding. Potential suicide attempters are often frequenters of outpatient clinics and have excessive hospitalizations and surgery [13]. Only a minority are ever admitted to psychiatric hospitals. The primary care physician who is aware of the demographic and clinical characteristics of suicidal persons will be able to identify the high-risk individual. Although most persons who share the demographic and clinical characteristics of high-risk groups will not commit suicide, large numbers of false positives do not preclude the value of early case finding.

Because of the close association between depression and suicide, it is important for the physician to recognize and treat depression as a means of preventing potential suicides. Instead of permitting depression to become a fatal complaint, physicians in Great Britain have practiced early intervention, which has been effective in lowering the suicide rate. Except for psychiatrists, physicians in this country generally have been less active in diagnosing and treating depression. There is substantial evidence that three-quarters of patients committing suicide had depressive illnesses, yet the diagnosis was rarely made in these patients [5].

ASSESSING AND TREATING DEPRESSION

Depressions can be conveniently categorized as follows:

1. Reactive depression—A normal response to a loss.
2. Psychoneurotic depression—Uses depressive symptoms in an adaptive way to cope with life situations. Brain physiology is presumed normal.
3. Endogenous depression—A disordered state of brain physiology.

Reactive Depression. To support the diagnosis of a reactive depression, an identifiable loss must have occurred. The patient's grief reaction should be appropriate to the degree of loss. The major signs of reactive depression are sadness, brooding, loss of appetite, and perhaps insomnia.

These are temporary, and within 3 weeks there should be little impairment of normal functioning. A reactive depression lasting more than 3 weeks without any sign of improvement should signal the presence of an underlying endogenous depression. The patient with a reactive depression requires reassurance. Minimal doses of a minor tranquilizer may be helpful.

Psychoneurotic Depression. The patient in a psychoneurotic depression frequently has a history of maladaptive coping behavior, such as alcohol or drug abuse. Symptoms including emotional instability, pessimism, hypochondriasis, irritability, anger, and dependency have usually been present for many years. Psychoneurotic depression responds quickly to therapy and then quickly relapses.

Endogenous Depression. The patient with endogenous depression may present with a multitude of symptoms, making a universal syndrome description difficult. The most marked cases may display psychomotor retardation, feel totally helpless, be preoccupied with somatic fears, sleep poorly, be agitated, and be unable to enjoy life. Common presenting symptoms include

1. Inappropriate fatigue or loss of energy—Fatigue is often described as worse on arising than later in the day. The patient often fails to fulfill the usual obligations.
2. Musculoskeletal complaints—Muscle contracture headaches with pain radiating to the neck, diffuse low back pain, or any pain that is out of proportion to physical signs is a common marker for depression. The pain usually begins after awakening, rather than the pain awakening the patient.
3. Nerves—Depression commonly accompanies anxiety. The anxiety of the depressed patient is manifested as irritability. Antianxiety medications may potentially alleviate symptoms. Any need for prolonged antianxiety medication should suggest underlying depression.
4. Gastrointestinal symptoms—When gastrointestinal symptoms persist with negative physical or radiographic findings and despite usually effective treatment, depression may be the

underlying cause. Long-term loss of appetite and energy is characteristic of depression.

5. Weight loss or poor appetite—Unaccountable weight loss, often accompanied by fear of a dread disease such as cancer, is a symptom of depression.
6. Sleep disturbance—Complaints of too little or too much sleep often suggest depression. Early-morning awakening is a symptom of two-thirds of depressed patients. Hypersomnia is a common complaint among teenagers.
7. Decreased ability to think or concentrate—This symptom is often not volunteered by the patient but may be readily admitted.
8. Loss of interest—The patient may complain that "nothing is fun any more" and may have a loss of interest in sex.
9. Thoughts of suicide or death—Fear of dying or a passive wish for death is a common symptom of depression.

When any of these symptoms persist for more than 3 weeks or is refractory to conventional treatment, an endogenous depression should be suspected. The presence of four or five of the symptoms occurring together as a syndrome will lead to a strong diagnosis.

In a relatively major departure from traditional beliefs regarding treatment of depression, some physicians are becoming increasingly aggressive in treating endogenous depression. They recommend that the diagnosis of endogenous depression is sufficient indication for treatment with tricyclic antidepressants. Furthermore, these physicians recommend that treatment with antidepressants be begun as soon as the diagnosis is made, even on the first visit. Because of the relative safety of the tricyclic antidepressants, there seems little justification for withholding pharmacotherapy. Many psychiatrists have traditionally recommended withholding drug therapy from the mildly depressed patient. It may be difficult to assess, however, just how mild the depression actually is and how destructive it actually may be to the patient's life.

It is understood and accepted that immediate and aggressive treatment of depression may result in some overtreatment. The consequences of delaying the indicated treatment, however, may be far more severe than the consequences of occasional inappropriate medication.

Immediate pharmacological treatment for endogenous depression is recommended once it is clear that the patient is not suicidal, psychotic, or suffering from a bipolar (manic depressive) illness. The treatment of choice is a properly planned regimen with one of the tricyclic anti-depressants. Noncompliance is the most common reason for therapeutic failure. Adequate patient understanding and preparation, including awareness of the side effects, will enhance compliance.

The tricyclic antidepressants can be divided into three chemical categories:

1. Imipramine and desipramine
2. Amitriptyline, nortriptyline, and protriptyline
3. Doxepin

Generally, amitriptyline and doxepin have the greatest sedating effect, but doxepin has less anticholinergic effect than amitriptyline. Imipramine is somewhat less sedative than doxepin. Protriptyline and desipramine have little sedating effect. The choice of an initial drug depends on which side effects may be desirable or undesirable for the particular patient. The side effects, though unpleasant, are benign except for aggravation of glaucoma and pos-sible increased morbidity in post–myocardial infarction patients. Commonly expected side effects are dry mouth (almost universal), urinary hesitancy (especially among the elderly), mild dissociation (transient), constipation, postural hypotension, ejaculatory or other potency disturbances, sweating, tachycardia, flushing, drowsiness, muscular "twitching," tremor, paresthesia, weakness, fatigue, headache, nausea, and heartburn. Common drug interactions are as follows: (1) Alcohol potentiates tri-cyclic antidepressants, (2) tricyclics potentiate anti-

Preventive Primary Medicine

Table 10-2. *Planning the Tricyclics Regimen for a Patient with Depression*

AGENT	PATIENT'S AGE	Initial	At end of 1 week	At end of 2 weeks reevaluate:	Weeks 3 & 4
Amitriptyline HCl (Elavil, Endep)	Under 55	100 mg 3 hr before hs (or a 2-3 day buildup to 100 mg)	150 mg 3 hr before hs	If excellent response, maintain same dose; check for side effects, reassure patient, review other diagnostic possibilities; review any lab work done; consider any changes to different tricyclics due to side effects. If 1. no response or suboptimal response, and 2. if diagnosis still correct, and 3. if side effects not prohibitive, proceed .	200-300 mg (if splitting dose, give most at night)
	Over 55	50-75 mg 3 hr before hs	100 mg 3 hr before hs		As much as clinical judgment permits you to give
Nortriptyline HCl (Aventyl)	Under 55	100 mg 3 hr before hs	See Comments		See Comments
	Over 55	50-75 mg 3 hr before hs			
Protriptyline HCl (Vivactil)	Under 55	20 mg in AM or 10 mg bid	40 mg any schedule		60 mg
	Over 55	10 mg in AM or 5 mg bid	20-30 mg any schedule		Rarely given to elderly in high dose
Imipramine HCl (Presamine, SK-Pramine, Tofranil)	Under 55	100 mg 3 hr before hs	150 mg 3 hr before hs		200-300 mg (probably splitting dose by clinical judgment)
	Over 55	50-75 mg 3 hr before hs	75-100 mg 3 hr before hs		
Desipramine HCl (Norpramin, Pertofrane)	Under 55	100 mg anytime	150 mg any schedule		200-300 mg splitting dose
	Over 55	25-50 mg anytime	75-100 mg any schedule		
Doxepin HCl (Adapin, Sinequan)	Under 55	100 mg 3 hr before hs	150 mg 3 hr before hs		200-300 mg, most at night
	Over 55	50-75 mg 3 hr before hs	75-100 mg 3 hr before hs		

At end of 4 weeks reevaluate:	Weeks 5 & 6 (if elected to proceed to max. dose)	SIDE EFFECTS*							COMMENTS
		Seda-tion	Anti-cholin-ergism	Sweat-ing	Orgas-mic dys-function	Cardiac arrhyth-mias	Appe-tite stimulus	GI re-actions	
If excellent response, maintain same dose for at least 2-3 months. If no response: 1. Again consider other diagnostic possibilities — psychosis, hypothyroidism, neurotic depression. 2. Utilize psychiatric referral. 3. If #2 not feasible, consider following options — A. Increase dose to maximum. B. Change to different class (as depicted here by shading) of tricyclic. C. Conduct a trial withdrawal; stop medications; see if patient gets worse, as a way of perhaps detecting subtle improvement, in retrospect.	Maintain maximum dose	4	3-4	0-1	0-1	0-2	4	0-1	FDA has not approved doses over 200 mg for outpatients. Most predictably sedating. Good when weight gain desired. Generally the best for agitated depressions, for early morning awakening, for older males (providing they have no BPH).
	See Comments	0-2	3-4	0-1	0-1	0-2	4	0-1	FDA has not approved doses over 100 mg, although no evidence exists that problems with nortriptyline are any greater with larger doses than is the case with amitriptyline and imipramine.
	Maintain maximum dose	0	3-4	0-1	0-1	0-2	4	0-1	Probably the most likely to cause stimulation, although this is debatable. May decrease appetite in some patients.
	Maintain maximum dose	1-3	4-5	2-4	0-2	0-2	4	2-3	FDA has not approved doses over 200 mg for outpatients.
	Maintain maximum dose	0-1	4-5	3-5	0-2	0-2	4	0-1	Most frequently used in older patients to avoid daytime sedation. FDA limits to 200 mg.
	Maintain maximum dose	3-4	0-2	0-1	0-1	0-1	4	0-1	Drug of choice when an anticholinergic effect cannot be tolerated, or when cardiac arrhythmias are a threat, or when guanethidine sulfate (Ismelin) must be used concomitantly.

*Scale of 0 (none) to 5 (severe).

cholinergic drugs, and (3) tricyclics inhibit guanethidine and reserpine. Otherwise the tricyclics are safe. The lethal dose is 10 to 30 times the therapeutic dose.

Table 10-2 outlines a suggested approach to planning a satisfactory tricyclics regimen.

OVERDOSE

Physicians can play another important role in helping prevent suicides. Of 122 suicidal deaths in St. Louis County, one-quarter were accomplished by ingesting an overdose, usually of a hypnotic [4]. The ready availability of a lethal amount of hypnotic has often been linked to incautious prescribing practices by physicians. Individual prescriptions of hypnotics should be restricted to no more than 10 to 15 times the usual hypnotic dose, usually a 2-week supply. Although this may not prevent a suicide, it may avoid facilitating one. Physicians should also consider dispensing hypnotic medications in individual or "blister" packets. The inconvenience of unwrapping individually packaged capsules may decrease the number actually ingested.

Summary and Recommendations

1. Depression—Depression, to be treated, must first be recognized. Probably the safest approach is for the physician to regard any depressed patient as potentially suicidal. Depressed men of any age and older depressed women are at greater risk. Physicians should ask every depressed patient about thoughts of suicide or a history of suicide attempts. Early and aggressive treatment of depression with tricyclic antidepressants is safe, is therapeutically effective, and may lower the suicide death rate.
2. Alcoholics—Alcoholics, particularly those who have suffered a recent loss, are at greater risk of suicide than are nonalcoholics. As with depressed patients, the physician should ask every alcoholic about suicidal thoughts or previous suicide attempts. The primary care physician may be influential in family counseling, offering greater support during the initial increased risk period or even, in extreme cases, suggesting hospitalization.

3. Previous attempts or threats—Both the threat of suicide and previous attempts, especially serious ones, place a patient in a high-risk group. The primary care physician is in a strategic preventive position because most patients who commit suicide are under a physician's care and because a majority of patients who commit suicide will communicate their intention. It is incumbent upon the physician to elicit this information.
4. Prescribing practices—Physicians should limit the availability to patients of lethal amounts of prescribed medication to help prevent suicide by overdose.

References

1. Beck, A., M. Kovics, and A. Weissman. Hopelessness and suicidal behavior. *J.A.M.A.* 234:1146, 1975.
2. Fawcett, J. Suicidal depression and physical illnesses. *J.A.M.A.* 219:1303, 1972.
3. McIntire, M., and C. Angle. Evaluation of suicidal risk in adolescence. *J. Fam. Pract.* 2(5):339, 1975.
4. Murphy, G. The physician's responsibility for suicide: An error of commission. *Ann. Intern. Med.* 82:301, 1975.
5. Murphy, G. The physician's responsibility for suicide: Errors of omission. *Ann. Intern. Med.* 82:305, 1975.
6. Murphy, G., and E. Robins. Social factors in suicide. *J.A.M.A.* 199:303, 1967.
7. Reich, P., and M. Kelly. Suicide attempts by hospitalized medical and surgical patients. *N. Engl. J. Med.* 294:294, 1976.
8. Robins, E., et al. Some clinical considerations in the prevention of suicide based on a study of 134 successful suicides. *Am. J. Public Health* 49:888, 1959.
9. Rosen, D. The serious suicide attempt: A five year follow-up study of 886 patients. *J.A.M.A.* 235:2105, 1976.
10. Shershow, J. The sometimes signs of suicidology (editorial). *N. Engl. J. Med.* 294:332, 1976.
11. The suicide profile. *Br. Med. J.* 2:525, June 1975.
12. Weissman, A., and J. Worden. Risk rescue rating in suicide assessment. *Arch. Gen. Psychiatry* 26:553, 1972.
13. Weissman, M. The epidemiology of suicide attempts. *Arch. Gen. Psychiatry* 30:737, 1974.

Index